MAGIC NURSE
BEDSIDE ARTIST

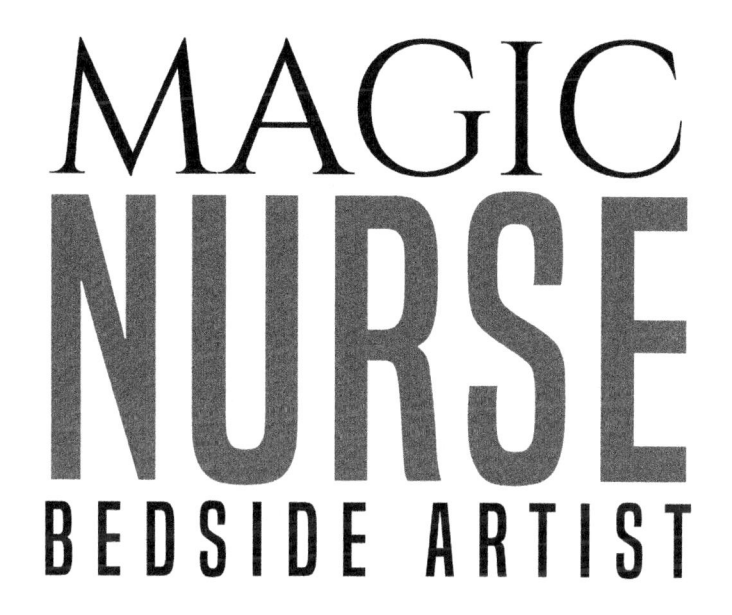

ROB DIVERS, RN
NURSE/CLOWN/MAGICIAN

Magic Nurse - Bedside Artist

Copyright © 2017 by Rob Divers, RN, Magic Nurse, LLC

All rights reserved. No part of this publication may be reproduced, distributed, or transmitted in any form or by any means, including photocopying, recording, or other electronic or mechanical methods, without the prior written permission of the publisher, except in the case of brief quotations embodied in critical reviews and certain other noncommercial uses permitted by copyright law.

For permission requests, write to the publisher at:

Magic Nurse, LLC
Attention: Permissions Coordinator
P.O. Box 1064
Euless, TX 76039

http://www.magicnurse.com/

Quantity sales. Special discounts are available on quantity purchases by corporations, associations, and others. Orders by U.S. trade bookstores and wholesalers. For details, contact the publisher at the address above.

Editing by The Pro Book Editor
Design by Indie Author Publishing Services

ISBN: 978-0-9986126-1-4

1. Main category—Nursing>Nurse & Patient
2. Other category—Nursing>General

Printed in the United States of America
First Edition

IN MEMORIAM

Magician and brother, Brett Wolf,
Your magic and friendship strengthened me.
May the Lord Bless all whose lives you touched.

DEDICATION

To my wife Darlene for picking up the pieces of a broken and burned out ER nurse. Through tireless faith and love you nurtured me back to health. Thank you for believing in every crazy idea I have. I love you beyond measure.

To my amazing children Christine, Catherine, and Andrew, I know it was a shocker when I became a clown after you all grew up and moved out. I hope you too will find your crazy shoes and run to your hearts delight!

To my first wife Gretchen, thank you for being a lifetime friend and a great mother to our kids. Our early years saw some terrible times and tragic losses, but our family never lost what mattered most.

To my hospital clown partner Robyn Sanford, your faith and courage is an inspiration to me. From the first moment you put on the red nose in that dark parking lot of St. Paul medical center, I knew you had the gifts for this loving mission.

My sincerest thanks to the many nurses who have found the magic in themselves. Your help in my journey has made it so deeply rewarding to be weird.

"Nursing is an art: and if it is to be made an art, it requires an exclusive devotion as hard a preparation as any painter's or sculptor's work; for what is the having to do with dead canvas or dead marble, compared with having to do with the living body, the temple of God's spirit? It is one of the Fine Arts: I had almost said, the finest of Fine Arts."

—Florence Nightingale

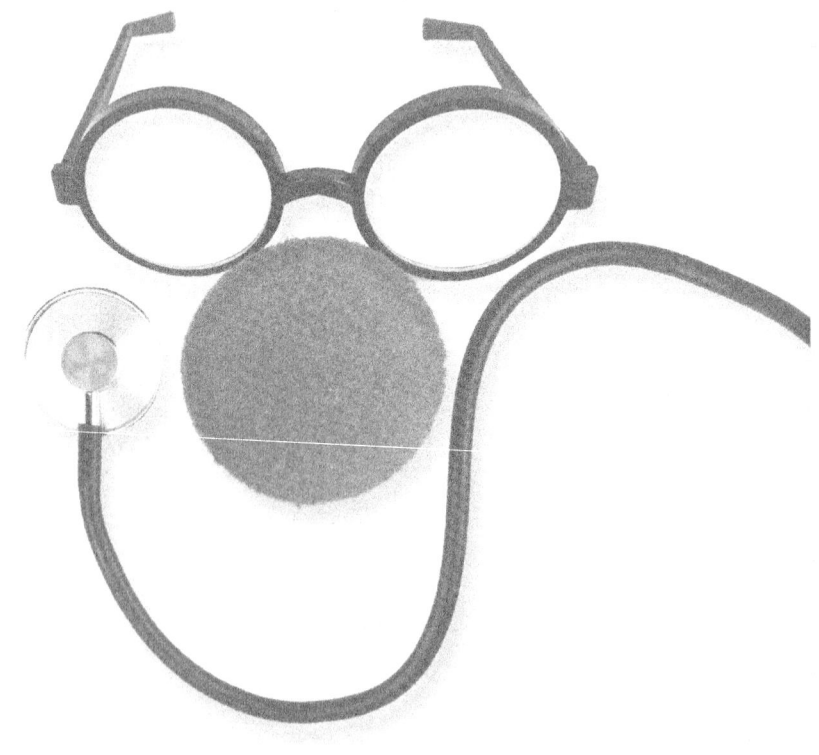

CONTENTS

Introduction ... 1

Part I: Motivation ... 5

Chapter 1
Lost Art of Nursing ... 7

Chapter 2
Do You Believe in Magic? ... 15

Chapter 3
A Star is Born ... 24

Chapter 4
Finding Your Patch ... 30

Part II: Mission ... 39

Chapter 5
Magic Nursing ... 41

Chapter 6
Clowning and Caring ... 49

Chapter 7
Hospital Magic ... 75

Chapter 8
Brett's Story ... 81

Chapter 9
Magic as Therapy ... 94

Chapter 10
Dream Doctor Project - Medical
Clowns in Action ... 101

Chapter 11
Flower Power: The Magic of a Rose ... 115
Chapter 12
Not Just a Nurse ... 123

Part III: Method ... 129
Chapter 13
The Clinical Artist's Toolbox ... 131
Chapter 14
Integrating Art in Hospital Systems ... 154
Acknowledgements ... 163
About The Author ... 167
References ... 169

INTRODUCTION

The primary mission of this book is to offer creative approaches to bedside manner. Whether you are a medical professional or visiting a friend in the hospital, using art as a caring act, is healing for everyone.

"Magic Nurse" originated as a nickname my patients and co-workers called me when I first started doing magic tricks in the hospital. I learned that the words represented something more—the vital importance creative connection offers in clinical experiences.

The words "magic" and "nurse" seem strange together. "Super Nurse" might have been a zippier title, and I know many nurses who are amazingly super! Super-Duper, in fact—cape and everything! Being a magic nurse, however, is more gentle and subtle, and easier to accomplish. No supernatural powers necessary.

The "Nurse" part is about nurturing and caring, and all the medical things we provide with the highest standards and integrity of the nursing profession. "Magic" is the good stuff you bring to the bedside while performing your medical functions. Magical bedside manner is as important to the care of patients as the medical tasks.

*Magic happens when you perform clinical
acts wrapped in creative expression.*

Having excellent bedside manner is the true art of healthcare. You perform real magic in those moments when you connect your humanity with your patient. Creative art, in whatever expression it takes, is an excellent vehicle for making warm and friendly connections.

Breaking the ice to make healing connections through laughter is a healthy exercise that improves breathing and circulation. Humor is so powerful when you use it to make your patient laugh or smile. Laughter releases endorphins and reduces blood pressure. Playful interaction is wonderful for easing the anxiety, fears, and loneliness of another human being. Illness is stressful enough. By improving the patient's environment, you also improve their mental and physical health.

If you have even the slightest desire to find a little more love for your nursing career, listen to your creative inner voice and follow your heart where it leads you. Injecting art into your work will result in greater joy for yourself and your patients. Have the courage to break down stereotypical expectations and share something special about yourself to those entrusted to your care. You are a caregiver, not a robot or a mindless machine. You may work in a complex system, but the rubber meets the road with your nursing shoes. Look deep into the eyes of your patients and connect with them where they are. Let them see who you are too. If you happen to have a clown nose on your face, even better.

> *Art is that part of being human where we express our emotional selves best. Caring is an emotional act, often coming from a place of love or duty to our fellow man.*

I made radical changes to develop a more fulfilling clinical practice for myself. I never would have believed I could be doing the work I am doing now. Over my lifetime, I have learned that magic is happening all around us. We just have to find it and claim it for ourselves.

Magic Nurse is a memoir wrapped inside a mission. It's my attempt at open heart surgery. Let's hope the patient and the message survives!

Patch Adams starring Robin Williams was an inspiration to me early in my career. The same is true for many doctors and nurses. This movie became a blueprint for many creative healthcare workers, inspiring the use of humor as a healing modality in their clinical practices. Those of us in the trenches of healthcare who focus on the person, not the disease, are exactly the kind of caregivers who should be overhauling our healthcare system from the bedside upward. The name Patch Adams has come to represent the intangible essence of creativity infused into joyful bedside manner. This concept resonates with patients today more than ever.

I found my "Patch-like" bedside manner through the use of magic, comedy, and music. I reached out to professional performing artists to learn, and to Dr. Adams in 2012 and became a friend and follower of his work. He is one of the best humans I have ever met.

I continued the study of hospital clowning and became good friends with many therapeutic clown professionals. Traveling to Israel in 2014, I learned valuable skills and methods from one of the world's best medical clown programs: The Dream Doctor Project. This unique organization has over 100 specially trained therapeutic clowns working every day in hospitals throughout Israel. These artists work in close collaboration with medical staff and add an immeasurable quality of compassionate care to patients young and old. I discovered a tremendous opportunity to combine the skills of performance art and medicine together and share it with medical communities at home.

I have asked two professional magician friends, Kevin Spencer and Michael Mode, to share a major piece of their magic journey with us. They offer some therapeutic effects of magic which are fantastic healing tools we can use every day. Any healthcare professional can apply a few of these easy to acquire magical skills and experience new ways to connect with their patients.

During the early phases of my journey as a clinical artist, I lost a close friend and magic mentor, Brett Wolf. He shared his gifts so generously in service to others. He was a true friend and brother, and I will never forget him. We worked on many ideas together, and he was the most intuitive advisor I had in this Magic Nurse mission. The most valuable art I know is the art of friendship. Being a friend to someone is itself a creative expression. It has the power to ease suffering and despair.

Many other performing artists, musicians, singers, clowns,

magicians, and Patch Adams himself were very helpful in completing this book. I learned how to combine art with my nursing work and discovered the powerful impact it had on my patients. Sharing art is the most loving and beautiful way to create healing patient-caregiver relationships. I found a magic ability that exchanged joyful energy in both directions.

Like you, we all have a life story that makes us who we are. I am sharing my experience so you may see how it happened for me. I hope my story helps you on your path.

Magic Nurse is about a creative restoration of joyful caregiving for all of us.

Is this possible? If you believe in yourself, anything is possible!

Are you ready to discover your inner "Patch Adams character" and find the artistic expressions that you enjoy most? If so, you will quickly see the opportunities to integrate your creativity at the bedside too. You will know when the time is right to use these skills because your intuitive clinical senses will reveal the perfect moments.

If you are already doing creative things in your practice, consider me a friend and let's swap ideas! I would love to hear from you. If my story inspires you, I would like to help you on your journey. I am happy to share all my best tricks!

Email me: DiversRN@MagicNurse.com

PART I: MOTIVATION

CHAPTER 1
LOST ART OF NURSING

"I am only one, but still I am one. I cannot do everything, but still I can do something, and because I cannot do everything, I will not refuse to do something that I can do."

—Helen Keller

FEW WILL ARGUE OUR NATIONAL healthcare system has never been good enough. The Affordable Care Act, aka Obamacare, was supposed to address the problems of providing access to everyone while finding ways to pay for it. The new law caused new challenges within the system while making old problems worse. Hospitals were stuck in the middle while still being expected to provide the highest levels of medical and technological care regardless of politics.

Medical facilities contain the latest scientific equipment, provide the latest surgical and diagnostic services, and deliver massive amounts of pharmaceutical products. The combination of all these technologies is what we think of most when we talk about our advanced medical system. Healthcare has become one of the largest growth industries in our economy. Today's hospitals are complex businesses, and their survival is dependent on profitability and the efficiency of the medical workforce.

There are new challenges driving nurses away from the bedside, where staff shortages have been a major problem for decades. Nurses have longer hours, higher acuity patients, and greater responsibility for larger numbers of patients. The demand for hospital beds is a strain on the entire system, putting the pressure on nurses to get patients off the unit as quickly as possible.

Inpatient hospital stays are shorter than in years past and patients are discharged faster than ever before. Time in a hospital bed is at a premium, and no one gets to rest at a hospital. We have learned to adapt to a systematic delivery of care by multiple organizations providing medical and pharmaceutical wonders of science in mass.

Though we call them patients, they are customers, and interactions with our clients have changed from a healthcare partnership to a customer service based transaction. As part of the Affordable Care Act, government reimbursements are now partially based on patient satisfaction data from surveys. Hospitals must work harder on customer service, becoming more like hotels, as patient satisfaction surveys have become a key driver in how healthcare is measured.

Nurse employment is projected to increase from 2.86 million in 2012 to 3.44 million by 2022 (according to the ANA, American Nurses Association). An estimated 555,100 RNs are projected to retire/leave the labor force, adding to the declining entry of new nurses into the profession. In 2008, the US was short 116,000 nurses. That is predicted to worsen to about 500,000 by 2025. The US will need to educate another million new nurses by 2016, which is 40% of the size of today's nursing workforce. [1]

These shortages are going to increase. Attraction to this profession is decreasing at the same time requirements for entry into nursing becomes more difficult. Hiring preferences have also changed in the last two decades to encourage entry level employment in nursing with a minimum of a Bachelor's Degree (BSN). This higher educational requirement has become a deterrent for many to enter into the profession due to increased costs of college. Thousands of working RNs who entered the profession years ago with less costly Associate Degrees (ADN) or Diploma certifications are systematically screened out of service in the larger hospital systems. Many large hospitals are requiring staff to return to school and earn a BSN degree to continue working in their current jobs, even though state requirements have not changed for nursing licensure.

A state issued RN license does not distinguish degree levels of competence. This push for BSN entry into nursing is a movement that is industry directed. I trust there are very smart reasons for this, but I happen to be an ADN in my mid-fifties with no plans to get a higher degree before I retire. I'd rather that seat is filled by a young nurse instead.

Diploma RNs are all but extinct, and hospital-based Diploma RN programs make up less than 10% of entry into nursing. Today there are less than 100 Diploma RN programs in the country, and this number is steadily shrinking.

Community and Junior Colleges across the country have produced the majority of working nurses in years past who enter the profession with an Associate's of Applied Science Degree in Nursing, or ADN. It often is the only affordable option for adult learners, single parents, and economically challenged students to become nurses. There is no difference in the bedside care whether a nurse went to a Junior College or University, all nursing programs prepare RNs for NCLEX exams and state licensure. Additionally, all nurses have access to specialized certifications to achieve even greater proficiency in their particular fields of practice like ER, OR, and Critical Care.

With 43.7% of hospitals and other healthcare settings now requiring nurses to have a bachelor's degree and 78.6% expressing a strong preference for the BSN, I believe disaster is creeping up on us. Our current nursing ranks show that only 55% of nurses working right now hold a bachelor's degree or higher. [2]

Caregivers are who patients rely upon to create the kind of healthcare they desire most, despite the increasing technological weight we carry. Patient expectations are naturally aimed directly at the professionals they meet in the hospital. We are the human face of healthcare when a patient arrives at our door, and this exchange is where it gets personal for patients. We as healthcare workers should take this more personal as well. Hospitals are only truly as good as the people who work there.

Thousands of treatment delivery processes existing within a hospital all layer in convoluted ways to make up the care delivery experience: diagnostics, lab specimens, blood tests, radiology, treatments, surgeries, therapies, social, financial, and spiritual consults. Assessments and procedures of every kind intertwine around each diagnosis to create an overall experience. With each process or medical element, there is an opportunity for the clinical employee to make a connection with the person in front of them. They look into what they perceive as the face of healthcare, searching the eyes of that technician, nurse, or doctor, to see if there is actually a compassionate human being looking back. Too often they only see the glow of a computer screen reflected back as the healthcare worker is clicking away on the keyboard while calling out a series of scripted questions from across the room. This is the new age of healthcare; it's a data-driven, technologically advanced model of care, and they tell us it is the best in the world.

It is easy to point at a system from the outside with its massive complexity and treat it as a huge problem requiring enormous fixes. The solutions—the best ones, I think—are going to come from much smaller adjustments on multiple levels, beginning at the hospital bedside.

At the front lines are nurses, RNs and LVNs, who stand at the bedside to assist patients every step of the way. Nurses attend their patient assignments day and night, providing whatever is needed. Emotional, physical, and spiritual aspects of care are all within our scope of practice. We are trained from the earliest traditions of our profession to be flexible in providing care and comfort when needed, at the proper times, being ever watchful to keep our patients safe. We use our hands to provide therapeutic touch for our patients. Nurses passively move limbs, moisturize dry skin, massage, bathe, and provide comfort by holding a trembling hand.

The patient-nurse relationship is a sacred trust borne from our deepest sense of humanity. In my nursing training, I worked with great nurses who were passionate about this profession. Compassion is the foundation of healing. Over time, these aspects of nursing conceded as technology crept steadily into patient interaction. Nurses had to adapt and accept the rapidly changing responsibilities technology brought. The profession has morphed into its modern, technologically dependent form, and when I look at the landscape of today's nursing profession, I believe we are in deep trouble already, and it could get much worse.

The increasing workloads on medical and surgical floors are stretching bedside nurses far too thin to offer any sense of job satisfaction. When nurses lose the love for their current positions, the temptation is high to jump to another hospital in hopes of better working conditions. It's a shell game, an illusion. It's tough everywhere.

Nurses are the target of non-stop marketing campaigns for employment. The shortage and demand for RNs have never been greater. Recruiters are constantly targeting us through direct phone calls and mail offers for job opportunities. Recruitment drives by hospitals and other systems sometimes offer outrageous sign-on bonuses in the tens of thousands of dollars, flashy new cars, and other perks to catch our interest in every major medical market. I get solicitations for jobs in my mailbox weekly, and I can see how a nurse might be just one bad day away from jumping to another facility with the same shortages.

It has become so competitive nationally that many state legislatures have adopted recognition of out of state nurse licensure to allow for rapid movement of RNs to work in multiple states. Travel nurses fill the most desperate shortages and take advantage of high paying assignments, receiving large bonuses with travel and lodging expenses covered. Hospitals are competing for the same limited workforce in local, and often national markets, while at the same time creating hardships for ADN and Diploma nurses. These competitive pressures are a weak solution for nursing shortages. We only need more new nurses to get in the business. If we can solve that problem, we'd have a good thing going. The situation gets a little worse, I'm afraid.

Seasoned nurses may be older and wiser, but we are not getting any younger. I am now 53 years old, and in our profession, nurses ages fifty and older make up 53% of working nurses today. That means over half of us will be shuffling off to retirement soon. I don't know about the other ADNs, but I am willing to stay as long as they'll let me.

Though the outlook for having enough qualified and competent nurses to care for us in the years ahead is bleak enough, other factors are helping to drive these numbers down. Bedside nursing as a destination profession is becoming more of a pit-stop as the requirement for higher education attracts nurses into advanced practices for higher wages and better working conditions by continuing education for a Masters or Doctorate in Nursing. Advance Practice Nurses often start in 6 figure territory and draw the most skilled nurses away from bedside nursing for the attractive salaries as a physician extender. Nurses moving into advanced practices are filling a growing void to help the ever-increasing physician shortages. Mid-Level Providers like Nurse Practitioners and Nurse Anesthetists help fill the gaps of doctor vacancies, which are also increasing. Having a BSN makes the next educational leap exponentially more attractive and sensible.

Most of the experienced bedside nurses you see today will be gone tomorrow, and the system we are currently building will not be better than the one it is fast replacing. It is diminishing from the inside. Caregiver time at the bedside is being reduced as a result of staff shortages and replaced, partly by the ever-increasing dependency on information technologies. Our new systems give us an incredible amount of medical data while robbing our patients of the human connection we once had.

Therapeutic touch is all but gone from our nursing practice as we have become data entry clerks for the information system. RN time at the bedside decreases as we are tethered to our computers instead. What is happening at the bedside of patients is where I believe our healthcare crisis begins. The bedside is where I most want to focus my attention as a care provider, to make the experience of a patient the best possible exchange in the lives of both. We are all going to be a patient in that hospital bed one day and will experience the business end of our healthcare system as a customer, but is that what we really want? Or do we want something better?

I am just one nurse who lives and works within the healthcare system we inherited. I cannot do big things to make the system better, but I can do small yet meaningful things that have great value. I can still care for my patients in a loving and compassionate way. Through the use of my personal creativity and healing intentions, I am a better advocate for my patients by treating my nursing practice as an art. The real art of caring for another human begins with connection. I cannot worry about the bigger problems. I can only get up in the morning and choose my day.

When I became a clinical performance artist, I found ways to express this caring and healing relationship by creating and including art at the bedside. Using arts like music, comedy, and magic, I bring a new therapy into my practice and add fresh delivery of care to the typical medical environment. A little bit of magic goes a long way to alleviate the stress of the healthcare system. Magic and humor reminds us of the wonders of our human experience and is a delight to the mind and spirit.

I discovered over many years of trying creative and unique ways to enhance the lives of my patients, the true magic I was looking for. The many happy and healing moments I create through art in the hospital has changed the course of my nursing practice. I cannot do much to fix our healthcare system, but I can make a little magic happen when it is needed most.

My sincerest hope is to help other nurses and healthcare workers discover their creative energy, use it to elevate their bedside performances, and enhance their clinical practices. If we can find new pathways to connect with our patients using performing art, we will restore the compassion we are losing in our profession. When we tap into our creativity, we heal ourselves in the process. Caregivers will have a better way to influence positive culture change within hospital systems. We each can inspire more compassion, joy, and connection in others by finding the light within ourselves first.

If we can give ourselves permission to be clinical artists, we will begin to heal our healthcare system from the inside. I believe it is Art and not Science that will take healthcare (and humanity itself) to the next revolutionary stage.

CHAPTER 2
DO YOU BELIEVE IN MAGIC?

"We do not need magic to transform our world. We carry all of the power we need inside ourselves already."

— *J.K. Rowling*

I was 28 years old, working as a sales manager at a car dealership when my father learned he had pancreatic cancer. At 52, he found out he had only months to live. We had a rough time in those terrible days while he battled that disease. I was thankful for how amazing his hospice nurse was as she cared for him in our home. She cared for all of us, actually, through the most difficult time in our lives.

Soon after my father died, I decided to go to nursing school, then chose the ER as my specialty. I wanted to help other families through dire circumstances like my family had been helped. I had the drive to confront human tragedy and was determined to learn how to handle every medical and traumatic assault that rolled through the ambulance bay. I could not save my father, but I wanted to save someone if it was possible to do so. I wanted to try.

I knew a career in the ER was a serious call as my eyes opened to the limitations of medicine and how fragile life is. Time is our most precious currency. In the first ten years, I had a front row seat to tragedy, trauma, and human suffering with great regularity. ER nurses see every kind of disease, injury, and abuse. I often felt my clock ticking, knowing it was statistically possible that I too could be scooped out of a burning, smashed automobile one day. There is no guessing who might be the next unlucky soul to suddenly be catapulted to eternity.

I often thought about my father and wondered if he would have lived a different life if he had known he would pull the short straw out of his pack of Camels and die of cancer at such a young age. I found myself measuring and forecasting my life by my father's life span, and this motivated me to waste less time doing things that did not matter.

I told my friends, "I value time more than money because my people don't live long."

Time is the only real treasure on Earth, and it spends very quickly.

With each year bringing me closer to that magic number 52, I accelerated my desire to make every day matter more by doing things I loved. I wanted to help people more, and I eventually learned how to combine my passion for performing arts with my nursing practice. Enhancing the lives of patients while filling my own time with the creativity I desired most seemed like the best way to go. I discovered the real magic of life by treating it as an art form. Being an artist at life means creating as many great moments as possible with the time you have; not just for yourself, but others too.

> *We cannot change the world by receiving things from it, but by what we give to it instead. In the end, we retain nothing of tangible value except the privilege of having given ourselves to others.*

Artists of every kind draw their most precious visions and ideas from within themselves. Through their art, they pass it on to audiences, observers, and listeners, delighting the senses of others. There is no better way to care for others than through the gifts of art, music, and compassionate presence. An extraordinary energy happens when an act of kindness is offered and received between people. It is palpable; some call it a "warm fuzzy." Feel good moments. When caregivers and patients share in this exchange, it produces real magic in the lives of both.

I believe the profession of nursing is built upon these "love thy neighbor" acts. Nurses care for the human family with a healing love of life.

John Lennon said, "Love is all you need." Imagine how much better life would be if we all took that more seriously. If we put more love into medical service, how much better could it be?

Do you believe in the power of love? I do.

I have a great friend, Shel Higgens, who I met while training in magic. He is a magician and street performer who went on to perform on America's Got Talent. He did dangerous things with a chainsaw and had many other great stunts, but in the early days, we worked together street performing locally. He performed a straitjacket escape while riding a tall unicycle. My job was to help him get safely on the unicycle and call 911 if the show did not go well. At the penultimate moment of his act, just before stepping over to a 7-foot unicycle from atop the ladder while strapped securely in the straitjacket. He looked out into the crowd, anticipation building, and shared a simple message: "Life is short…do what you love, I do, and I hope it shows!"

Shel is living out his love for others through his art too. We both appreciate a great verse in Hebrews, 13:2 that says, "Be not forgetful to entertain strangers: for thereby some have entertained angels unawares." We rarely get to see how our actions ripple beyond our knowledge to affect those around us. But we know deep down that it matters very much that we do these acts of service anyway. Angels come in all shapes, sizes, and colors. Some even laugh at our jokes.

Do you believe in Angels? I do. I've met some. Many of them are nurses!

When I began doing magic for my patients, I was surprised at how great sharing this art was for both patients and families. The gratitude, the smiles, and the tearful hugs from parents thanking me for giving their child a unique moment were the most important kinds of moments I had ever experienced. I had to continue replicating those magical moments in as many other lives as I could. I had never given medicine or performed a procedure that did more for my patients than when I created magic for them. I discovered a new way of being a caregiver! I became a Clinical Performance Artist! I used magic initially but soon learned that all the performing arts had powers for healing.

To medical professionals who are not yet believers, take an assessment of your clinical life and see if there is anything missing. If you lack a sense of joy or creative fulfillment, it might be time to explore new possibilities. I hope you find even one small action you can add to your clinical practice that will give you as much enjoyment as I have in mine.

My intention is to inspire you to take a closer look at creative possibilities you may not have considered before. Great gifts of discovery are waiting. Once you find your superpower, and the impact it will have for your patients, you may experience a decrease in your stress and start having fun again. Creating joy works for patients and staff! Do not take yourself too seriously on this journey; you must allow yourself to let go a little bit and imagine a new character for yourself. When Bruce Wayne and Clark Kent become Superheroes, they wore their underwear on the outside. We can take some fashion risks too. I bring extra clown noses and a giant pair of underwear with me to every hospital visit. It amazes me how easily I can get medical professionals to put on the red nose, climb inside the world's largest pair of underwear with me, and parade around a medical unit. Instant comic relief helps an entire floor, staff and patients alike.

Your creative passions are valuable parts of who you are. Real magic power comes from the uniqueness we each have. Believe that your creative gifts are worthy of sharing with others. Whatever you do for fun is a good place to find your superpower.

For me, it was a love of music, clown comedy, and sleight of hand magic that found its way into my clinical career. There are endless artistic possibilities, though. Performing arts has universal appeal, and it is up to each of us to discover our relationship to it. It is far too easy for adults to put aside their personal passions for the arts to become professionals in business and medicine. Professional business-minded people are just sleeping artists who put their creativity on a shelf like an old toy they outgrew as they became grown-ups.

You can still do art and be a professional;
it will actually make you better at it.

Wherever you may be in your life at this moment, you have the power to change anything you desire. Start walking toward your goal, and you will arrive. Sometimes we find ourselves in places we never imagined we would be. We may also carry regret from choices we made along the way. It is never too late to discover your art. You can reach back into your childhood and rescue any dreams you left behind.

Whatever your passions were in youth while your ideas were magical is where you will find your superpowers again. Your inner child lives on, making silly faces at you when you aren't looking. From my experience as a medical clown, I met many playful children still residing inside adults in ICU beds. Our inner child is still in there and wants to find us again too. There is always time for joy, even if time is short.

From behind the red nose, I discovered the ability to connect instantly with kids and adults in many hospitals and communities here in the USA and around the world. Language and cultural barriers disappear for the clown, and the game is about playful connection. What I learned through clown art is that you can help a person play again, joining your inner child with theirs, especially if you have an extra clown nose to share so they too can feel the freedom and fun a red nose can offer. I always have enough new clown noses for everyone, and it's great to see the instant transformation in others when they wear the red nose. It is a healing experience for the patient and me. My batteries get recharged every time!

When I do magic for my pediatric patients, their parents are along for the ride too. Caring for a child in the hospital is a family affair. As I perform magic tricks for children, parents experience wonder through their child's eyes. The family dynamic is wonderful. When parents take their kids to Disney World, the grown-ups have just as much if not more fun than the kids.

My favorite use of magic was to provide an instant distraction that takes a person out of their anxiety or fearful emotional place through an entirely impossible diversion. The effect is immediate and has a lasting influence. I carry at least ten magic tricks in my scrub pockets every day I work as a nurse in the hospital. Unlike the clown, when the wearing of a red nose telegraphs the knowledge that there is a clown on the way, a magic nurse or clinical magician has the element of surprise on their side. You as the clinician can decide when a little magic might help a situation and begin with a simple offer.

"Would you like to see a trick?"

When the answer is yes, you open up an opportunity to connect and create a fun experience. I perform three magic tricks in less than two minutes that will have a lasting impact on the patient's experience. Even a single magic trick taking only seconds can have kids talking about magic for weeks.

Magic as a therapeutic modality is another aspect this art form can be used to empower patients. By having specific magic tricks you can perform, then teach to those patients who want to learn magic for themselves, you can introduce an activity that will provide therapeutic value long after you have gone. Project Magic and Healing of Magic are great programs we will talk about later. You may be surprised how this unique aspect of magic contributes to physical and cognitive therapy. I get excited just thinking about it!

Performing magic in the hospital preceded my venture into medical clowning. Combining these arts added momentum to the clinical impact as each appealed to my sense of child-like wonder, putting my brain to work imagining impossibilities.

*Okay, so what does all this talk of magic
and clowns have to do with you?*

These are just examples of my personal superpowers. I bring this stuff to work with me, making it part of my practice as a pediatric nurse.

Trust me! You can do it too! Find your superpower and take it with you to your job!

It was a little scary for me at first, but I did it anyway. Was I concerned about what the other nurses and doctors would think of me? Was I worried about getting in trouble? Certainly. This behavior was not the normal execution of regular nursing duties. I wrestled with the idea, made a good risk-benefit assessment, then stuffed my pockets with magic tricks and did it anyway. I performed a little magic trick whenever I saw it would do some good for my kids. I found that it did a lot of good and soon took off as a new thing for me.

Thankfully my co-workers appreciated what I was doing, and we all had fun entertaining our patients. When doctors started calling me in more frequently to do magic for their patients, I began to realize the real power of this art. I taught several doctors how to perform tricks too. Even with this level of acceptance, performing bedside magic was not officially sanctioned. I never actually ran this by anyone for approval. Magic was just part of my personality and bedside manner. Patients and families loved it! Today my use of healing magic is widely encouraged, and we are finding ways to expand our creativity in more clinical areas.

I invite you to explore for yourself what you can do to make your clinical practice more fun. Find a creative thing that is joyful for you and share it with your patients. But don't just stop there. Challenge your co-workers to do the same. If you have to spend long days working with stressed out staff, it might be time for a magic and comedy consult on your unit!

You can be the catalyst for creative change, and it is needed now more than ever. Our healthcare system has become so chaotic and impersonal; it desperately needs an infusion of creativity and compassionate human connection. Science has held the reigns of our medical delivery approach, and it is time for art to find its way into the action.

Do you believe in magic?

Your journey belongs to you, and I hope you will take the road less traveled too. I've met many remarkable people along the way. Art is life, and if we are in the business of saving lives, I think we would improve our healthcare system considerably if more medical professionals became "Clinical Performance Artists."

TOP 10 REASONS TO BECOME A CLINICAL PERFORMANCE ARTIST

1. Work will be fun.
2. Patients will love you.
3. It's the best cure for stress and burnout.
4. Creates the joyful job culture you desire.
5. Positively affects satisfaction surveys.
6. Life will be a daily adventure.
7. Invigorates creative inspiration in others.
8. Therapeutic applications are endless.
9. Increases compassionate creativity.
10. Changes our healthcare system from within.

CHAPTER 3
A STAR IS BORN

"All the world's a stage, and all the men and women merely players; They have their exits and their entrances, and one man in his time plays many parts, His acts being seven ages. At first, the infant, Mewling and puking in the Nurse's arms."

—William Shakespeare, As You Like it.

From the moment of our birth to our last breath we are performing the act we call life. Our mere arrival into the world of light is a joyous event met with a media frenzy of cameras and videos. Even before our debut, our parents can get a sneak preview with 3-D sonogram technology to see if we are going to be a leading man or lady. We hit the world stage as a child star, and our fans delight in every burp, fart, and smirk with amazement. Parents applaud our every little movement and expression, even delighting when we produce something interesting in our diapers. We are a miracle to behold as our first typecast role as a human baby begins. That first bar is set pretty low for us; we are born a child star. Soon enough we'll be learning lines.

A mother's love is the first magic any of us experience. From her body and soul, she creates life with magic given by God Himself. She nurtures us, shows us what dreams are, and infuses us with courage to become explorers and creators in the world. She is our first contact with the source of imagination, wonder, and possibility.

For the first several months, we are observers of our natural processes and learn about hunger, satisfaction, and relief of discomfort. We marvel at the faces of our parents making sounds and expressions that comfort us. Everything we do is naturally entertaining to them, and we, in turn, smile back at their silly, loving mugs.

My earliest childhood memories were glimpses of discovery. Adventures were illuminating around me in every direction. Always nearby, a soft hand appeared at times necessary to adjust objects within my reach. A young magician's first lovely assistant is his mom who is always on cue, setting the stage for every routine. Our first music is hers. Costume changes, all her. She appears at the right times and for all the right reasons.

Soon we learn to respond and become imitators of what we see and hear; we imprint these expressions and begin to adjust our responses to suit our desires for attention. Our natural born talents develop, and we imitate and improvise as we mimic whatever catches our attention. We laugh and cry a lot. We take on the subtle traits of others. This imprinting is the beginning of the lifelong roleplay we adopt to create ourselves and the personalities we become. We are characters of our own creation through the help of our parents first, and then others follow. The progression of influences becomes infinite from there.

Pre-school years in early childhood was a magical time for me. I plugged into television so intently; I swear I passed through the glass and lived on Sesame Street. Mr. Rogers neighborhood was the next street over, Romper Room and Captain Kangaroo were also favorite stops. Our Zenith console brought the world to me, and I traveled in starships before I ever rode a bicycle. We had only four channels on the television back then. Difficult to imagine that now. I spent many hours with the Flintstones and the Jetsons, time traveling from prehistoric past to unimaginable future. I am still waiting for flying cars.

"All the world's a stage" from Shakespeare's classic play *As You Like It* has stuck with me from my early childhood. I am not sure when I first heard it, but it gave me an early understanding of life and society. It provided a context I could easily grasp that helped me relate to everything. Blessed with a wild imagination, I found play-acting a favorite activity. Mimicking TV characters was like a reflex I couldn't control. I was mesmerized by television and absorbed everything I could from the parade of images and stories it brought. I could sing all the catchy jingles, and sitcom theme songs have stayed with me over a lifetime. Bugs Bunny and friends taught life lessons. I learned about conflict from Natasha, Boris, Moose, and Squirrel. Sadly, I realize now my important social skills came from the animated lives of barnyard animals.

I learned a lot about culture and society from Looney Toon characters. My first exposure to classical orchestral music was through cartoons and the conductor Leopold. My introduction to Opera and Shakespeare delivered through parody by Elmer Fudd, and Bugs made me passionate about the classics. Learning how to prepare hasenpfeffer was the highlight of my culinary education too, although pop tarts suited me just fine. Cartoons are treasure chests packed with hidden knowledge about ourselves and our world. A clown can find endless inspiration from them. I return to them often for material and ideas.

As a teenager, I was naturally attracted to acting and was active in our high school and community theaters. I shared those glory days with many creative friends as we all experimented with our artistic gifts. I could talk and sing like Kermit the Frog back then and loved music theater. I played guitar and sang in a musical trio called Pastel with great friends Cathy and Rick. I wanted to be an actor/singer when I grew up. That was the dream anyway. I adjusted my aspirations and sought reality roles with steady paychecks as I matured and needed to feed a family.

I believe we indeed are "merely players" in the world, and I have fashioned my approach to every job I ever took as a dramatic role. I studied my part, learned the lines, and performed in the best manner that I perceived the role should play out. I don't know exactly why I have always thought this way, but it seemed logical and worked best. You pass the audition, study for the role, and perform.

With each career advancement, I prepared for it with intensity to be the best I could be in the role. I worked a variety of restaurant and retail jobs at first, then worked my way into better gigs. I was commissioned as a bank security guard once and carried a Smith & Wesson .357 magnum, which I thought made me cool like Magnum PI. In truth, I was more like Barney Fife.

I eventually landed a better role and found a Ford dealership to be my first big break at age 21. I had a great ten year run as an improvisational performer in this outdoor amphitheater we called a car lot. I considered auto sales to be the best paying acting job I would ever hope to have. But when my father was diagnosed with pancreatic cancer, I left that role to be cast in a medical drama that continues to this day.

I found that with proper character preparation and careful study, actors deliver performances that satisfy and delight audiences (or bosses). When you seek perfection in a role on stage or in life, you work hard, study hard, and deliver your best performance. It's an act of service in its most creative form, involving every aspect of mind and body.

Every actor develops their personal interpretation of their roles, and I believe people genuinely do this in their lives too. I think people play many parts, whether they admit it or not. A person can have many outward characters in public, and yet the actor beneath, the true self, can be entirely different. I look for the clues in a person's outward character that points to the human actor within. The comedy and tragedy masks are just two extremes of a thousand masks people can wear. It's important to look beyond the surface to consider the human person living inside. It takes an effort to maintain masks, and some actors are splendid in their roles.

Some folks are natural improvisational artists who create themselves in every moment, no masks needed. What you see, is what you get. They are the most fun to connect with because they usually lack a filter and are making everything up as they go along. I love improvisation more than anything because it is a free flow of ideas with endless possibilities and no fear of failure. Life is improvisation. We might not appreciate the improvisation skills we already have, but we actually use them every day.

Let's take a look at our hospital stage through a theatrical filter. The hospital is our Globe Theatre! It is a microcosm of the world where tragedy is more often out of balance with comedy. It's a magnificent performance center where actors are cast from both the highest and lowest status of society, yet work on the same stage. Off stage, cast and crew live worlds apart but come together to perform our unique medical drama and share the limelight together.

The Divas (surgeons) make grand entrances and execute their command performance with perfection. Principal characters (doctors, nurses, therapists) perform leading roles driving the action, creating tension, resolving conflicts, and enter and exit on cue. The supporting cast (housekeepers, food service, materials, engineering, medical records, et al.) make occasional cameo appearances but work mostly backstage in practical invisibility, making the stage function properly and keeping props clean and moving. Casting calls and rigorous auditions by HR discovers new talent while stage managers (hospital administrators) are responsible for keeping the entire theater operating. Admins manage the venue and make sure the lights stay on. They keep a close eye on the front of the house; ticket sales, audience response, and show promotion are all necessary. The show must go on! Our lives depend on it.

The hospital is also the place where most of us happily begin and sadly end our lives, making entrances and exits onto the world stage. Arrivals occur in the Labor and Delivery department typically, though we have caught a few immediate deliveries in cars and hallways for those players who missed their cue and came too early.

Departures, final shows, and season finales are frequently found in the ER where tragic and often sudden exits occur with high drama and surprise plot twists. The ICU can also be a place where many leave our stage, yet many others do return and give grand encore performances, staying in the limelight with us a little while longer. Sometimes the sequel is even better.

We healthcare workers are always performing, whether we are providing care to patients or interacting with other members of the hospital cast. Since we are performing as clinical characters already, why not go that extra step and become clinical artists. We can enjoy more thoroughly the parts we play and provide blockbuster experiences for our patients!

The actor inside made me a better nurse once I found how to access my creativity again. You can find yours too! Becoming a clinical performance artist improved my effectiveness and increased my enjoyment of caring for patients. I studied sleight of hand magic from the best magicians I could find to prepare for my magic nurse character. Whatever character you wish to play has resources available you can tap into as well. And it's never too late to watch cartoons for inspiration or just to find your uninhibited, playful side again.

Learning a new artistic skill or reviving an old one is liberating and rewarding. You owe it to yourself to restore your creativity.

Performing magic at the bedside helped me considerably, but I had only scratched the surface of the healing power of performing arts. My hope is to assist you to become a clinical performance artist and learn why it is just as important an enhancement of your personal health and professional well-being as it is a readily available healing joy for your patients!

CHAPTER 4

FINDING YOUR PATCH

"You treat a disease, you win, you lose. You treat a person, I guarantee you, you'll win, no matter what the outcome."

—Robin Williams as Patch Adams.

I<small>F YOU'RE READY TO DIVE</small> into the idea of what creative and compassionate care can look like, and you have not seen *Patch Adams* with Robin Williams, you should watch it as soon as possible. Get your tissues ready; it has some tender moments that could make your eyes leak.

This movie introduced new and unconventional ways to connect with patients. People recognize humor at the bedside as "Patch Adams" moments because it had a lasting impact that continues to resonate with people today. Many medical professionals have been motivated to become better caregivers by this movie. It was an inspirational and influential film for those who made their career in medicine, and I was one of those people.

Patch Adams was released in theaters December 1998 and had an excellent reception, making it number one its opening weekend, then stayed at number two for four weeks. The movie was loosely based on a small part of the life of Dr. Hunter "Patch" Adams during his time at medical school. It was there he discovered and championed a way of approaching medicine in creative ways that defied the established hierarchy in medical school. In the movie, he risked being expelled for his unorthodox methods. He redeemed himself in the end by the support of the nurses and patients whose lives he touched. Robin Williams expertly played the role of Patch and captivated the hearts of people the world over, even though the film itself received mediocre reviews. Roger Ebert, Chicago Sun-Times, claimed it was too "syrupy," giving 1 out of 4 stars and calling it a "shameless tear-jerker." Siskel & Ebert both gave "two thumbs down" on their television series.

The critics may have missed the indirect impact this film would have among medical people. I've heard many people say, "Oh, you're like Patch Adams," whenever I did magic for them. I noticed that quite often the name Patch Adams became a description assigned toward any playful behavior of caregivers in medical settings. This movie was the only example people had for this atypical bedside manner. I get the impression there is a huge desire for more of this type of creative expression from healthcare workers. The idea is that medical care delivered with humor is a welcomed concept that benefits both clinicians and patients. Patch Adams started his personal revolution in healthcare long before any of us knew who he was. His movie began to open our eyes to the possibilities he imagined.

The video was available for rental the following year. I did not see it at the box office as I was a busy ER nurse in those days. When I eventually saw the movie, it set in motion a profound change in me that would influence the course of my life. It was not that the film was that profound, but what was happening in my life that forever linked me to Patch, his movie, and the clinical direction I would eventually take.

Do you still have those tissues handy? It gets rough here for a bit.

My father Bill Divers passed away in 1992 at the age of 52, after a brief battle with pancreatic cancer. My mother Judy, who was a traditional stay at home mom and housewife, was devastated when her whole world crumbled at the loss of her high school sweetheart and husband of 32 years. She had shared her life with her best friend and raised four sons with him. As she worked through her sadness, she found comfort in using her loss to help others who also lost loved ones.

My mother went on to start a nonprofit organization called GROWW: Grief Recovery Online for Widows and Widowers. It was an online website that provided chatrooms hosted by other compassionate volunteers to give peer support for others experiencing grief. Open 24/7, this became her life's work to honor my father's memory and find meaning in her loss.

This mission gained worldwide reach in the early days of the internet. (remember AOL and dial-up modems?) GROWW found friends and followers everywhere the internet had a foothold. My simple stay-at-home mother quickly became well-known in grief work, and local groups of supporters assembled and organized in many places across the country. They organized special weekend support group meetings and called them GROWW gatherings. People who supported each other in online chatrooms could finally meet and fellowship with their peers in person, strengthening bonds of friendship. My mother was treated like royalty at these gatherings and often received acclaims and awards for her work. People loved her, and she never got used to the attention or the status her supporters treated her to.

I remember a catchy phrase the hosts used back then: "WWJD" meant "what would Judy do?" In the chatrooms, visitors were received with warm cyber hugs that looked like this: (((((((((((Judy))))))))))))). Even stoic men with their bottled-up emotions could find a safe and anonymous way to grieve with peers who shared their stories too.

After seven years, in October 1999, I was invited to share in an event in Oklahoma City at a GROWW gathering where my mother was to receive a Governor's Commendation and honorary citizenship for her work with the people there in the years following the Oklahoma City bombing in 1995. During my visit with her that late October weekend, my mother and I were amazed at how much of a deal people made about her. She never felt like she was anything special; she just loved people and knew how to listen and share and connect like any good person would do. I was so proud of what she had accomplished, turning her loss into such a positive work. She was a real superhero, and love was her super power.

She had a cough that weekend and was taking a round of antibiotics for a new diagnosis of bronchitis. She was feeling a bit run down but didn't let it show, and I suggested that she go in for a chest x-ray when she got back to Orlando to check things out. I drove back to Dallas and was never more proud of what my mom was doing in the world. I was her nerdy, quirky son growing up, and knew very well how loving and nurturing she was. Seeing her treated like a celebrity for these traits was heartwarming. By the following Wednesday, I got the call from Mom that her x-rays showed a significantly large tumor in her right lung. Things were not going to turn out well.

It was a few days before I was able to arrange the time off work to fly home. It was early November, chemotherapy and radiation treatments were already underway, and she was losing her hair by handfuls when I saw her next. My father's battle with cancer had lasted several months before his fight was over, and we were ready for this fight too. We knew the drill and were doing everything with hope and positivity. While I could only stay a few days this visit, I was making arrangements to be as much help as I possibly could.

After our morning trip to the cancer center for radiation treatment, my mother had the Patch Adams movie rented at home and wanted us to watch it together. We settled into a quiet afternoon starting with lunch and talked about everything. After lunch, we played the tape. She had already watched it once but wanted to watch it again with me because she loved it, and she wanted me to love it too. I did.

In her grief work with GROWW, she had many kind and beautiful words of comfort she shared with people, and the online community was just as generous with their love and support in return. Everyone contributed their compassion and understanding, and sometimes that was all that was necessary. One of the ways they dealt with anniversary dates of deaths was to refer to them as "Birthdays to Heaven." After a proper time, the hurt and sadness of grief would give way to a fond remembrance and joyful anticipation for when we too would have our birthday to heaven and be reunited again forever!

Living with cancer became a powerful tool for Mom during her last weeks as she wanted to convey her intuitive understanding of the end of life as a time to love and share joy while we're heading for that big heavenly birthday bash in the sky. There were things in the Patch Adams movie that resonated with her strongly, and Mother wanted to be sure I understood them and would do something about it in my nursing practice.

In the movie, Patch encountered a woman near the end of her days who was not eating well. When he met with her, she revealed how she always wanted to swim in a big pool of noodles. Patch made that wish come true for her, and the scene that delighted my mother most was the one where she and Patch joyfully swam in noodles together.

"That is how I would want to spend my last days. In a hospital like that!" she said, smiling. "It would be fun!"

The next part of the movie that left the strongest impression on mom, and the reason behind her marching orders to me specifically, were represented in the scenes about the angry dying man with terminal cancer who threw things at the nurses. She had seen for herself how a strong man was brought down low by cancer. She loved and comforted my dad through all the suffering he endured. As a loving wife who did everything she could, she saw the beauty in how Patch helped this man. She immediately appreciated how using humor as a healing tool for a dying man was a valuable means to help men like him face death with strength, honesty, and integrity. The ability to laugh at ourselves in our nakedness, weakness, and imperfections is a liberating experience. No one had spoken to the dying man in a way that connected him honestly with his fate, and Patch found a very simple key to unlocking the grip of anger. He connected with his patient and give him comic relief so he can find peace and comfort without wasting what little time he had left being isolated by his anger.

"I want you to be a nurse like Patch Adams," Mom said. "You should go work for him!"

Mom and I spent that week together and soaked in as much as we could out of our time. She was insistent that I assume her role as President of the board of the non-profit, and to see that Jim Kennedy, her dear best friend and GROWW partner, would continue her mission as Executive Director after she was gone. We both knew how this was going to end, and we did not pretend otherwise. We faced the truth in love, but I thought we would have more time than we did.

I was wrong.

Three weeks later, on December 5, 1999, while working in the ER at Cook Children's Medical Center in Ft Worth, I got the crushing phone call from Jim that my mother died in her sleep while taking a late morning nap. Mom was 56 when her birthday to heaven came. It took me a long time to compose myself before I could drive home from work that day.

So you can appreciate how precious my last visit with my mother was in retrospect. It reinforced the importance of always taking full advantage of every living moment we have to spend with people. As an ER nurse trained in adult and pediatric trauma, I saw too many sudden endings to ignore this terrible truth. I rekindled the pangs of my personal losses with every family I met in the course of my work and connected with my patients' families as best I could to get them through the first moments of their loss. The drama of these events stays with you forever, making every loss part of our reality as nurses. We are all human. I've seen a few miracles in the ER also, but never enough to erase the sense of profound loss that sad departures leave behind.

That precious afternoon my mother and I watched *Patch Adams* together was the passing of a torch of love that Mom wanted to continue in the world. She knew there was a compassionate and creative soul dedicated to service at the core of my being, and wanted to be sure I was experiencing joy while doing it.

My mom's Patch Adams wish was a seed sown on fertile ground. Mother knew the actor/singer artist was still dormant behind the medical mask of her son playing the role of ER nurse. She had a means to communicate that directive to me though the example set in Patch's movie. Yes, the movie was a real tear-jerker, shameless in fact, but important lessons in life, humanity, love, and care were shared. It resonates with patients who know this movie too. People want their medical providers to be compassionate humans. The movie inspired many medical folks to seek better ways to be better healers. The concept of "Clown Doctors" also became a newly energized possibility, and medical clowns as a profession began to gain some real interest as a result of this movie.

The real Dr. Adams, now in his 70s, continues his mission today. He creates friends all over the world who want to help him build a free hospital in Hillsboro, WV at the Gesundheit Institute—a place where the entire staff is happy, funny, loving, cooperative, creative, and thoughtful, and caring for others is a privilege. The free "hospital" began in 1971 as a group of twenty friends, three of whom were doctors, opening their six-bedroom home to the public for free healthcare. Over its twelve-year history, an estimated 15,000 patients received care. Patch's dream of building a full-scale rural hospital began there too. His dream was presented in the movie, and in reality, is still an ongoing mission for the real Patch Adams. Robin Williams did a great job playing the character of a younger Patch and shared a small part of this dream in the film. May his memory be a blessing.

Dr. Adams made it his life's work to teach medical professionals, clowns, and others to be better at loving each other in friendship to create healthier communities in the world. For the past 32 years, Patch has personally touched the lives of hundreds of thousands of people on clowning missions around the world. Patch made each individual he encountered feel as though he had a real friend in whom they could rely on for love, truth, honesty, and friendship.

Patch encourages this experience as an open invitation to anyone who desires to learn compassionate clowning to join him on mission trips. Many doctors, nurses, medical students, artists, and clowns from around the world join to experience the healing powers of clowning for people in harsh, distressed situations like politically hostile countries, impoverished regions, and even war zones.

The art of clowning is a powerful method of reaching and connecting with people for whom just a little human compassion can be a giant relief from despair. Patch teaches by lectures, workshops, and by example, leading at least six clown missions a year. For those who have journeyed with Patch, the experience was a priceless lesson in life.

After my mother's death, it was thirteen years later that I would finally reach out to Patch Adams and explore my personal understanding of what his work meant to me. It was my mother's desire that I would seek him out, and I was always drawn to fulfill that wish and learn what I could from the man behind the movie. My clinical work continued in those years between, and the stress of working in trauma slowly added increasing weight to the losses in my life. I eventually decided to withdraw from emergency nursing. I took a position in pediatrics and found the magic again. Magic and a Mission!

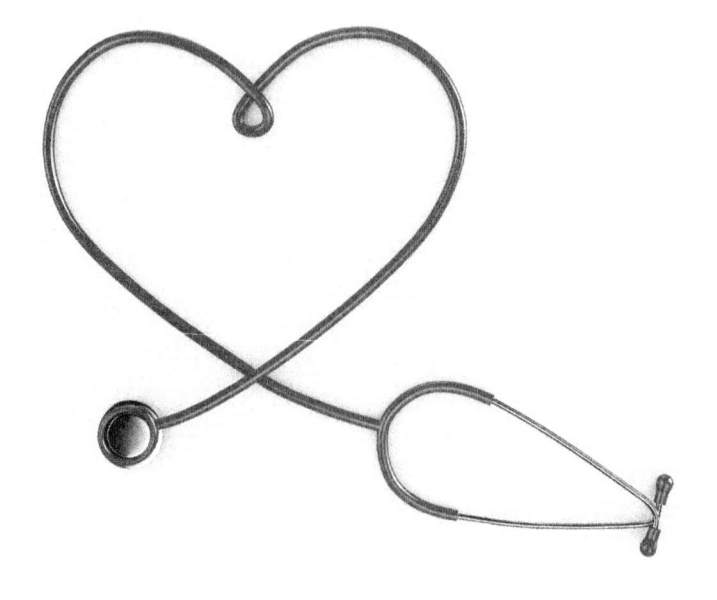

PART II: MISSION

CHAPTER 5
MAGIC NURSING

"Everyone has creative potential. Creativity involves using your imagination and inventiveness. Your unique expression of yourself is your creativity...Creativity can be magic when visiting people who are ill."

—*Patch Adams, House Calls*

I HAVE BEEN A REGISTERED NURSE since 1994, having left a 10-year career in auto sales to learn what I could about medicine following the loss of my father. Medical shows like *Emergency*, *ER*, and *Doogie Howser* were my motivational guides in medicine. It was a significant leap of faith, but if Doogie could do it, I could too. I desired to be more helpful to people than offering choices of leather versus cloth seats, power windows, locks, tilt, and cruise.

As an ER nurse, I obtained specialized certifications and maintained competencies to practice in trauma and pediatric emergencies. Having the knowledge and experience to deal with every possible medical emergency was empowering. Nursing skills become expert level by necessity very quickly. There is a standard training technique doctors and nurses are familiar with called: the "See one, do one, teach one" method. With constant changes in surgical techniques, new medicines, and treatment methods, and annual CE (continuing education) credits required to maintain licensure, medical professionals are in constant learning mode.

Those who work in this field become hardened and rely on proper training and knowledge of protocols to operate on such an intense level. Eventually, this challenging work takes its toll on people. Burnout is a common problem among emergency room staff. "Burnout" might be too gentle a word; PTSD may be more appropriate in some cases.

I began to feel the effects of this stressful, fast-paced work after several years of seeing the same traumatic events replayed over and over again. A continuous parade of horrific injuries rolled through the ambulance doors. Heart attacks, strokes, overdoses, stabbings, gunshots…you name it, we've seen it. Having a front row seat in this theater of horrors, in full 3D and Dolby Surround Sound, is not something you can endure forever.

The show does not end, however. The credits never roll. You personally have to decide for yourself when enough is enough and walk out of the show.

For many medical workers, coping with constant stress is difficult. Burnout, drug and alcohol addiction, failed relationships, negative attitude, and impatience and hostility towards an unrealistic and non-compliant public are just some of the manifestations. We all have met at least one grizzly mean doctor or nurse, right?

Personally, my happy fuse was very short after ten years in the emergency room. I had little sympathy for coughs and sniffles and an even lower tolerance for stupidity. Don't even get me started on child abuse. Staying professional in the presence of an abusing parent made my head explode. I had a poor attitude and developed a quick temper. I needed a break. I was suffering from burn out but failed to realize it. I will spare you the details of the troubles at home, but after a failed marriage, it was a miracle I survived and dug myself out of the rubble that was my personal life. A complete spiritual, personal, and career makeover led to my lifesaving marriage to Darlene! Remember those

Angels I mentioned before? She is one of them! (This love story will have to wait for the movie.)

I transitioned completely out of trauma nursing and moved into non-emergency pediatrics. Thankfully, this step quickly led to a revival of my spirits, and I was able to recover my compassion for nursing again. Removing myself from the front lines was the beginning of recovery. With my tour of duty over, I discovered something magical about the privilege of working with kids. The life and death stress was gone, and I had more time to spend with my patients and families. It did not take long before I was happier and enjoyed my work again.

Job stress is a well-known problem in critical care areas. Be open to considering another clinical specialty if you have lost the joy of your work. Surgery, Pediatrics, or Psychiatric nursing might be a good place to chill out for a while. You may even try Home Health on for size. There are many other places you can be a nurse, each with its own unique experiences and opportunities. Critical Care nursing skills will be welcomed in any specialty area you choose. Be proud of your service, and move on to the next gig. You have done your time in the grinder and made a difference. Thank you for your dedication. Now let a younger class of nurses set their hair on fire for a while.

Working with kids is great; they are just a whole different kind of people. Children will tell you exactly what's wrong, they recover faster than adults, and a popsicle makes a lot of things better quickly. I enjoyed making my kids laugh, and the more I played, the better a nurse I became. Making fun happen for kids in the hospital is challenging, but there's always a place for it in pediatric care.

Working in a children's hospital, I discovered my love for magic again. I had a few distractions ready to help ease the boredom for a patient or to alleviate anxiety. It was so easy to do, and it worked like magic! Performing magic soon became my favorite way to motivate and cheer up my patients.

Many patients lived at the hospital for several months during long periods of treatment or multiple corrective surgeries. My patients deserved fresh material from their nurse-magician regularly, which made my magic repertoire grow. Once you get something like this started, it takes on a life of its own. I have been using magic regularly at the bedside of my patients for more than a decade now, and it has proven to be the best nursing skill I have ever discovered for treating the blues, boredom, stress, and anxiety. Before long, I was carrying over a dozen close-up magic effects in my scrub pockets at all times.

Patients and co-workers alike started calling me "the magic nurse," and that title stuck. I also frequently heard parents and families say "Oh, you're like Patch Adams!" Time and again I heard this, and was fascinated that Patch's name was used so often to describe this type of interaction.

The power of a simple magic trick is a very unexpected and sudden game changer for patients and their families who are absorbed in coping with their healthcare situation. When an amazing visual effect takes place right in front of your eyes, especially when it's performed unexpectedly by a nurse in the hospital of all places, whatever anxiety or troubling mood instantly melted away. We connect in non-medical related roles as magician and spectator, momentarily transported out of the medical environment through magic, and turn fear into cheer.

What an awesome way to take a small mental vacation from our troubles! This playful diversion from reality benefits both patient and caregiver, allowing a shared experience for a better healing relationship. By sharing art, we are treating the mind and spirit of the person, instead of only treating the patient.

Before long, the pursuit of magic took a more definitive intensity when I felt it was time to elevate my magical techniques to a more expert level. Just like with the emergency skills I once learned, I felt that the same degree of expertise should apply to magic. No patient of mine deserved any less. They have already paid a high price to be in the hospital, and I felt they should experience the best magic I could give. So I embarked on a search for professional level magic training, and I found it!

While my magic library exploded with volumes of classic magic books, I also found an online website and magician's forum called The Magic Cafe at http://www.themagiccafe.com/. This forum was perfect for connecting with other magic enthusiasts throughout the world, both professional and hobbyist alike.

In ancient times, closely guarded secrets handed down from master to pupil in a mentoring relationship ensured the craft of magic remained protected. The crafts of carpentry, masonry, metalworking, music, art, and philosophy were also among those higher skills, as well as early medical practice. Do you remember Mickey Mouse in *Fantasia* as the Sorcerer's Apprentice? Thankfully, studying magic is not quite as intense as that.

Magic has no degree plan or residency program to follow, and there are many styles and forms of this performance art that can be studied. Performance magic may range from close-up sleight of hand, card magic, coin manipulation, classic street magic, parlor magic, stage illusions, and now television. What is not self-taught through books and DVDs is found in those trusting friendships that form when a student of magic seeks a teacher to instruct them. I found several top magicians who graciously gave of their time and resources to assist my education over the years.

The mentor and student should each be compatible with the other, for these types of relationships tend to be long lasting. Mentors are skilled masters who are genuinely interested in seeing their students succeed. The student is responsible for being attentive and respectful, often doing tedious side work as repayment. Medicine used to be like this, and many similarities continue today. Many interns might say nothing has actually changed.

My first magic teacher, Christopher Lyle, is a dear friend and a great instructor. He has always been a magician, never had a "real" job, and is a working professional who supports his family by performing magic. He guided my skills to a level I would never have accomplished on my own. Christopher's performances were great, high energy and exciting. I desired the same perfection and quality of performance for my work in the hospital.

Another great magician I found was Justin Styles, who is an award-winning magician from New York. Despite never having seen him face to face, with a single act of generosity he demonstrated to me the true heart of service many magicians have. What he did for me blew me away, and I will never forget his kindness.

One of my favorite magic effects is accomplished with a unique magic prop that allows the performer to produce a glowing red light on the fingertips at will and manipulate it in surprising ways. This routine usually was my opener in most of my magical bedside performances, and I wrote about the experiences I had with this prop in the online forum. Justin sent me an entire case of the commercially marketed props to give to the kids in the hospital. I soon realized that as I became more acquainted with the professional magic world, that there would be many other great men like Justin who were also eager to share what they could to help others through magic! As a nurse who does magic, I was very fortunate to discover how much help there would be for me within the magic profession.

In the Dallas/Ft. Worth area, there is a very active magic community, and many professional magicians originated from there. I eventually became a member of the Dallas Magic Club and was inducted into the Society of American Magicians by the Society President, Dal Sanders, who has been a great friend and advising supporter of my magic nursing. The Dallas magic community plays host to many great lecture opportunities from the world's top magicians, and the availability of professional education is the best. (outside of Las Vegas, of course)

The pursuit of knowledge, in any discipline, begins with the inspired desire of the student. I did not have to look long nor far before I found all that I needed to grow. Classic magic books published over hundreds of years, professional mentors, educational DVDs, enthusiast communities, and professional societies became my means to learn this unique performing art.

I cannot forget to mention the best resource of all: A brick and mortar Magic Store! Magic shops are harder to find than in years past, but they are the best place to start your mystical journey. One session with a magic demonstrator will hook you. Visit Derek Kennedy at Magic Etc. in Fort Worth, and thank me later. Walking into a magic store may be all you need to feel your inner 8-year-old come back to life!

Over a relatively short time, I became more confident in my magic skills with the help of generous magician friends. Their support and enthusiasm fueled my aspirations at every step to bring the best magic I could perform for the benefit of my patients.

The art of Magic Nursing is just doing something special out of your personal bag of tricks to be a comfort to another human being. I found sleight of hand magic to be a great vehicle to find this deeper connection, but there are many other arts that we can use for the same purposes.

Being a nurse has its scientific side, but the holistic nature of care must consider every aspect of our human nature: physical, mental, and spiritual. Sharing artistic gifts connects people on a more human level. When I share magic as a caregiver, my patient and I find a connection and share in playful relief for a moment. Magic is a way to extend kindness and friendship that enhances and improves supportive care. The same would also be true for music, comedy, clowning, storytelling, and puppets.

Artists of any type can find the healing aspects of their art to share in clinical settings. The nurse who finds their art within themselves will discover the most powerful healing tool they will ever have. It takes desire, courage, and commitment to excellence, just as it did for the completion of your medical education to become a therapeutic artist. You will not earn any new credentials that will be recognized by the medical world, but you will be adding something far more valuable to your practice. You will have greater passion and joy in your career and new abilities to share with your patients. Applying magic, or any artistic skill, to your clinical practice is the key to finding the joyful talents that will add real magic to your life as well as others. Having these tools available and knowing when and where they will help a situation is how you as a professional will make the biggest difference in the lives of your patients.

You still have super powers you may have long forgotten. Take a quick moment and pretend to be eight years old again. You will find them. Sometimes you have to go further back than you realize. It's worth the trip, I promise.

Allow yourself to be different. Patch did, and he is still inspiring joyful and loving change in the world. He also invites you to chase your wildest dreams! Write him and ask anything you like. He makes himself available to anyone who wants to reach out for a hand in friendship.

CHAPTER 6

CLOWNING AND CARING

"Unite your mission with your personal, perpetual experience of the miracle of life. Celebrate and be thankful that you have it together enough to step out of your selfish self, and have the opportunity to give yourself to others and to the world."

— *Patch Adams, M.D., "Gesundheit!"
with Maureen Mylander*

On February 7, 2012, I wrote Patch Adams a heartfelt letter sharing my story and the impact his movie had on my mother and I back in 1999. I told him how she wanted to swim in the noodles and spend her last days in his hospital. Patch sent a handwritten letter back twelve days later with a signed copy of his book and an invitation to come with him on a clowning mission that year.

Patch wrote, "I too was a product of such a mom."

He shared how the swimming in the noodles experience came about and told a sweet story of how in 2010, he recreated that experience for a 78-year-old nurse from Switzerland who had accompanied him on numerous clowning missions to Russia. I was so excited to have made a connection with the real Patch Adams and thrilled to take up his offer for a clown mission trip.

For over thirty years, beginning in 1985, Patch has been taking clowns around the world to distressed communities and hostile locations to relieve the suffering and despair of people in hospitals, prisons, war zones, refugee camps, distressed villages, orphanages, and psychiatric institutions. (fun places, huh?)

I signed on for a clown trip to Costa Rica in September 2012. The time spent in preparation for this trip was critical because I was about to spend a solid week immersed in humanitarian clown work with the most inspirational clown doctor of our age. I needed to get ready to be a clown nurse. So I went to clown school in May of 2012 to prepare.

As fortune would have it, I was acquainted with the founders of a fantastic clown school. Dick Monday and his wife and clown partner, Tiffany Riley, taught European theatrical style clown arts in a school called New York Goofs. What made this work out so perfectly was that this school originated in New York and for the first time, they held a "Maymester" Clown intensive near me at the University of North Texas Campus. The timing and location were right, so I signed up for clown school. I was going to be a medical clown with Patch Adams, and who better to train me for that experience than a clown instructor team who also worked in the clown doctor program at Dallas Children's Medical Center. [3] Called Funnyatrics, it is one of the few professional medical clown programs in the country.

New York Goofs clown school was a fantastic weeklong introduction into the finer aspects of performing as a theatrical clown. Sharing the stage with other clowns and theater students from around the country, I learned how to work with clown partners in the rhythmic beats of comedy, improvisation, physical movement, circus skills, dance, and classic clown gags and skits. Receiving a pie in the face is not for the faint-hearted, nor is correctly taking a pratfall. I did not realize how much technique is required to spit water in a steady stream or a bursting spray at your clown partner, depending on the comic intention. Clowns can be really messy.

I discovered my inner clown while drawing on my early high school years as a drama geek to appreciate the theatrical aspects of clown art. In traditional theater, an actor prepares for a role for a brief run of the show. When it's over the character dies at the last curtain call. Not so with a clown. Clown character is yours to keep! It's the alter ego you make for yourself and enjoy for as long as you desire.

Bruce Wayne became Batman, and I was carefully creating my very own superhero too.

The journey of discovering your clown requires reaching back to your childhood memories to remember how your child brain responded to the world, then returning those discoveries to the awareness of your character. Cartoons help to restore that child-like logic we still possess, though buried deep inside. I cannot say enough about the therapeutic value cartoons have for clowns. If you get a chance to observe a group of 4- to 6-year-olds watching cartoons, they will show you how to think and act as a clown.

I was motivated to improve as a performer by focusing on theatrical principles and worked to create a clown character I would use in public and medical venues. I studied everything I could find on clown arts, history, theory, and practice as I designed my performing clown character Tater, the tramp clown.

The Tramp or Hobo clown is a character that first appeared in American circuses as a parody character reminiscent of the train-hopping vagabonds. Tramps and hobo clowns are of American origin, and I appreciated that American connection. The great and unique characteristic of the tramp clown is the ability to share a range of emotions in their performance. Not all clowning is zany fun and games, as tramp clowns share their empathy for sadness too. If the Tramp had one superpower, it is the ability to recover from any adverse circumstance that he faces. There may be sadness, but it is not defeating by any means.

I chose the name "Tater" in tribute to the famous American tramp clown Weary Willie, Emmett Kelly's iconic clown character. In his autobiography *Clown*, Emmett wrote:

"In school, the kids called me 'The Irish Potater' or finally, just 'Tater,' and it used to make me sore." [4]

I liked the name and the connection to the great American clown. I was also frequently teased in school and could embrace the idea that Tater would be an empowered and positively hopeful character, in spite of his lowly status and poor fortune. Tater the Clown works for food doing magic, music, or anything that is necessary to chase your blues away. Tater took upon himself whatever remaining troubles I was still carrying around and made me a completely happy person again. (Thanks, Tater, I owe you one!)

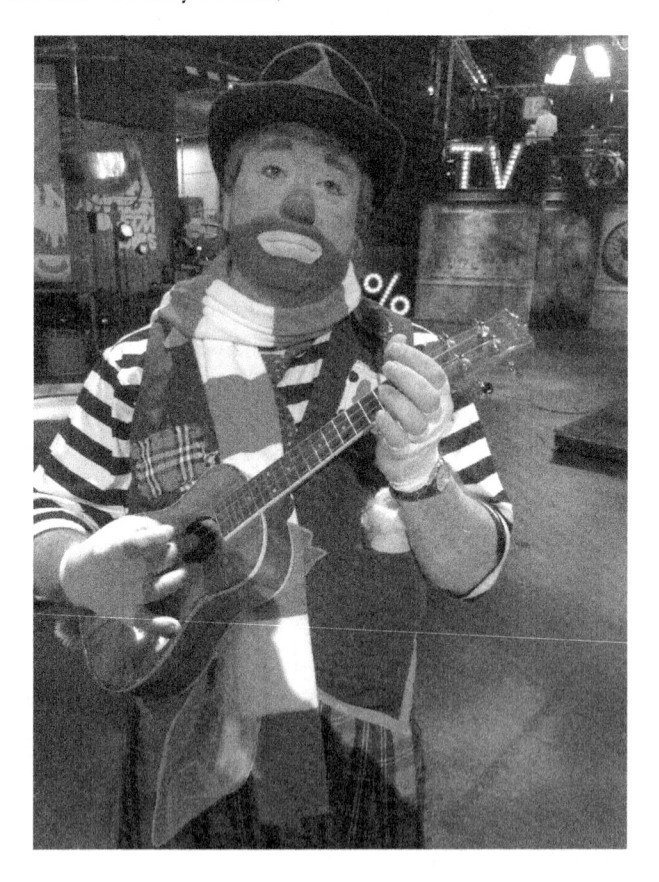

Another famous tramp clown that influenced the birth of Tater was Red Skelton's Freddy the Freeloader. [5] Being a TV clown, Red Skelton was much more visible to the TV generation of kids. I had the thrill of appearing once on *The Blaze* and met Glenn Beck before a State of the Union address. Tater was hired for a political purpose that day, and it was a good paying gig. Glenn gave me the highest compliment after the show, saying I reminded him of Red Skelton's clown. A comparison I certainly did not deserve, but it thrilled me to know that Tater made a good impression on Mr. Beck. [6]

At the end of clown college, a new clown is referred to as a "First of May," which is a reference made to newly trained circus clowns in their first season of a circus tour that starts in the spring. I was now ready to take my new clown into the world, prepared for a special mission. No protection of a circus tent, no peanuts or cotton candy for me, thank you. My clown was trained for warfare. I became a clown to bring compassion into dark, difficult, and dangerous places for healing purposes. With my red nose and clown shoes at the ready, it was time to bring the good fight to the enemy. Fear, anxiety, loneliness beware: clowns are coming to kick your butt! It was go time for my clown mission!

September came and I was ready to join the 2012 Clowning and Caring mission to Costa Rica with Patch Adams and his team from Gesundheit Institute. We were told to dress in clown attire for the entire adventure to get used to the idea of encountering the world through our clown at every step in our journey, and that included airports. Imagine the thrill I had when facing the TSA agent from behind a clown nose as he gave me the stink-eye.

"What's that red thing?" he said, pointing to the nose. (maybe a plastic explosive?)

"It is a disguise," I told him as I flashed a smirk.

The other agents nearby laughed, but stink-eye kept his composure and waved me through the body scanner without the need to pat me down or perform a cavity search, or whatever those guys do for fun.

Arriving at San Jose International, I met up with a few more clowns from around the US and other parts of the world. We were easy to spot due to our mismatched and colorful clothing. Clown noses helped identification considerably as we found each other in the terminal. We met Dario, Melanie, Elizabeth, and Jacob from Gesundheit near the baggage claim and waited for the others to join us. Before long, many of the clown travelers had assembled, and introductions ensued. Our eclectic group of artists, doctors, nurses, actors, social activists, business professionals, and lovers of a peaceful world would fast become friends. We bonded and learned from each other during this trip, each of us filled with passion for humanitarian relief work and excited about the opportunity to work with Patch Adams. We would soon share creative moments of connection in some very hostile conditions. Many of us continue our friendships, corresponding regularly to this day.

We settled into a modest hostel near downtown San Jose, which was our home base for the week. There were about 22 clowns in our group from around the world, with six guides from Gesundheit. On the first morning, we had an orientation meeting to prepare us for the first of several clown missions we would experience. We became more acquainted with each other and began to gel as a cohesive group. Herb and I were the only RNs, but there were two young ER Physicians and Radiologists, Eberhart and Danielle from Rio De Janeiro and Joaquin and Danella from Puerto Rico, and Carlos, a medical student from San Juan.

We had a variety of non-medical clowns too. Compassionate artists from around the world made our eclectic group well-rounded in talent and experience. Paloma from San Antonio was a medical translator. Shelly was a theater director and actress/playwright. Gem, a beautiful young actress from Scotland and Alex from Australia, were amazing. Julianna was a medical student from New York who had been on other trips with Patch. Lisa, a free-spirited artist, and Richard, a businessman, were also from New York. A mother and son team, Cate and her multi-talented teenage son Jamie came from California.

Another Kate traveled from Germany to join Patch's clown mission. Sadie traveled from Nova Scotia with her friend Elizabeth. Elizabeth, a gifted poet, was the first ever wheelchair bound clown to go on a mission trip with Patch. A sweet young lady with a heart for service, she never let her physical limitations stand in her way. Elizabeth would have some extraordinary moments on this trip. I stayed close to Sadie and Elizabeth throughout our time to assist with mobility.

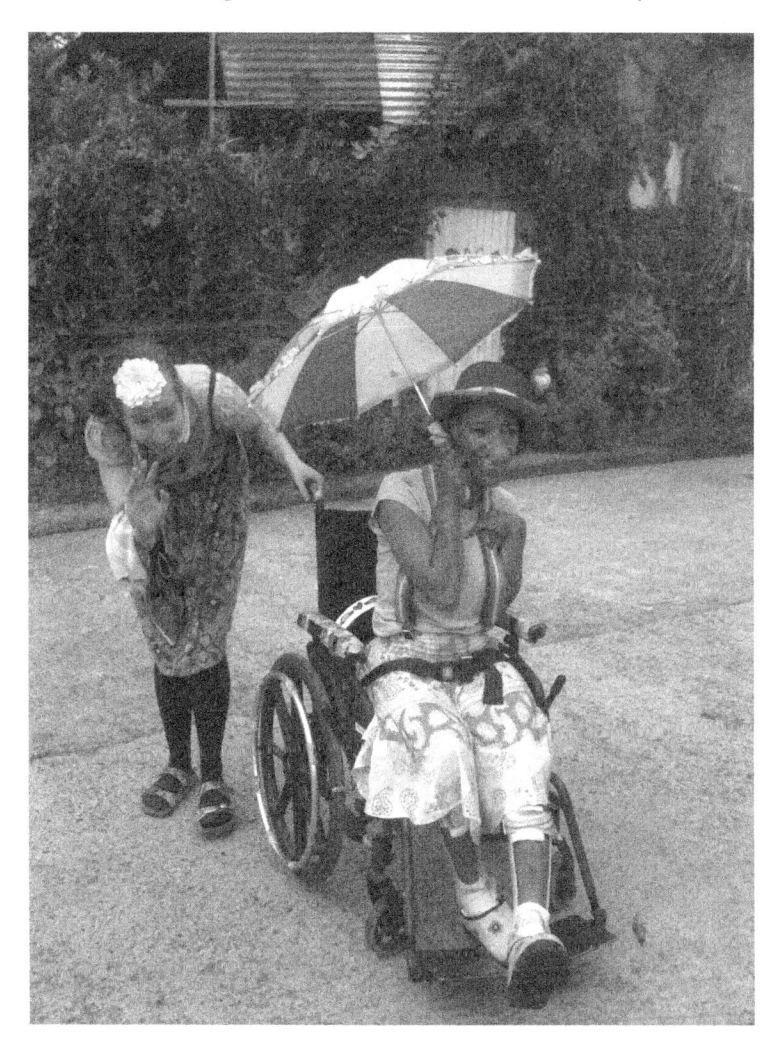

On the bus rides each day, Patch held a briefing on that day's mission and shared experiences of previous trips to prepare the team. He made a point to visit with each of us individually and in small groups. Getting to know us was just as enjoyable to him as it was for us.

"I would like to become friends with all seven billion people on the planet," he said.

Watching him engage people wherever he happened to be, I felt he was well on his way. Patch was gracious everywhere he went, drew many to him, and made everyone feel valued.

The first day, we traveled by charter bus to a severely distressed and poor community called La Carpio, a district outside of San Jose consisting of primarily Nicaraguan refugees who escaped the civil war of the 80s and 90s. It was considered the most dangerous and poorest concentration of about 35,000 settlers who made their home between a landfill and two polluted rivers. Plagued by high crime, unemployment, and destitute conditions, this troubled place became our outdoor theater. For two days we would enter this community and connect with them in dirt streets with open sewers and scattered trash. La Carpio became our playground when she was not busy being a violent and dangerous ghetto.

We made our way street to street and house to makeshift house, splitting up into smaller bands of clowns to embrace this community and play with its children. We sang songs, danced with them, and celebrated together as we expressed our friendship and love. A little goes a long way in La Carpio, and we had moments of connection that surpassed any experience I had ever known up to that day. We brought our hearts into this distressed place and bridged the divide from our reality to share in theirs. This place was desperately poor and full of trouble, but when the clowns came, there was a temporary release from the grip of fear, violence, and poverty. The circus had come to town.

Of all the moments I cherished, there is one that stands out the most for me. Sadie, Elizabeth, and I were making our way to see a special girl we learned of who also had cerebral palsy and was wheelchair dependent. When we found the corrugated tin shelter where she lived, her mother brought her out in a wheelchair fashioned from two bicycle tires and a white plastic lawn chair. When her eyes met Elizabeth's, the explosion of joy was incredible. A beautiful clown in a wheelchair came from a faraway land especially for her!

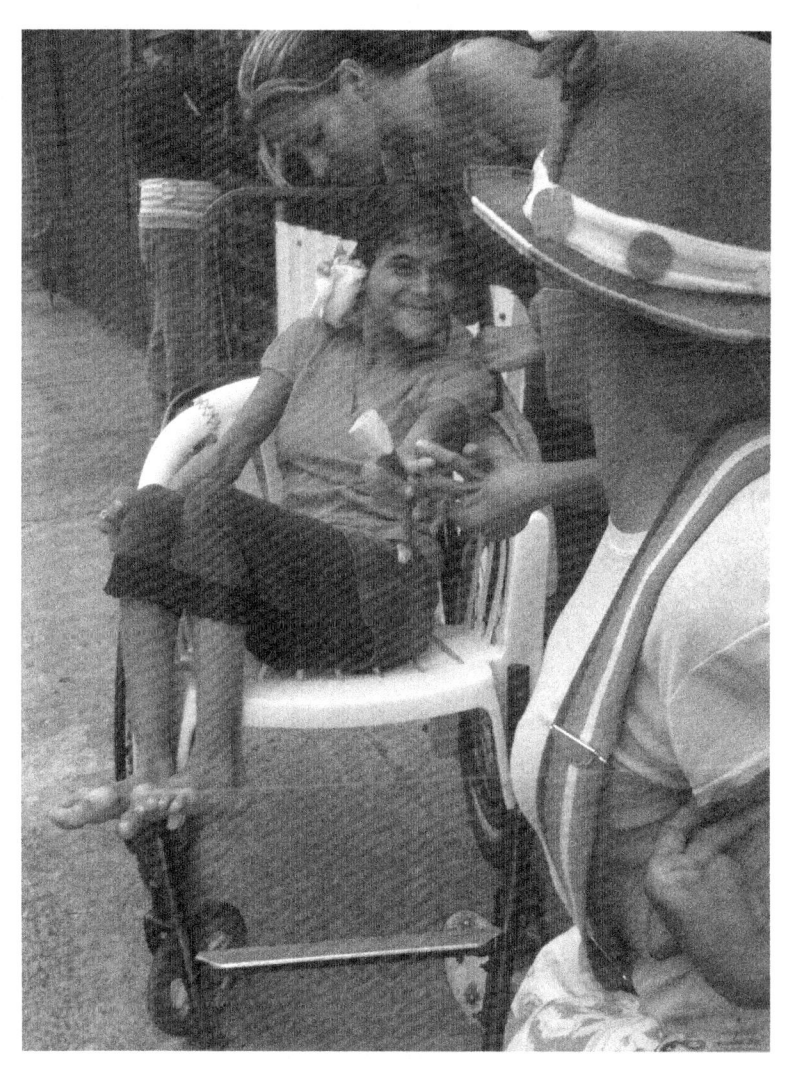

The young girl beamed with such intense smiles it brought joy filled tears all around. We never wanted this moment to end. Elizabeth saw her new friend as the sole reason she traveled so far to discover her clown. I quickly made a paper flower for Elizabeth to give her, and she placed her clown hat and a nose on the girl, and she became a clown too. I still get tears when I think of that encounter and those precious minutes watching those two sharing this very special visit together.

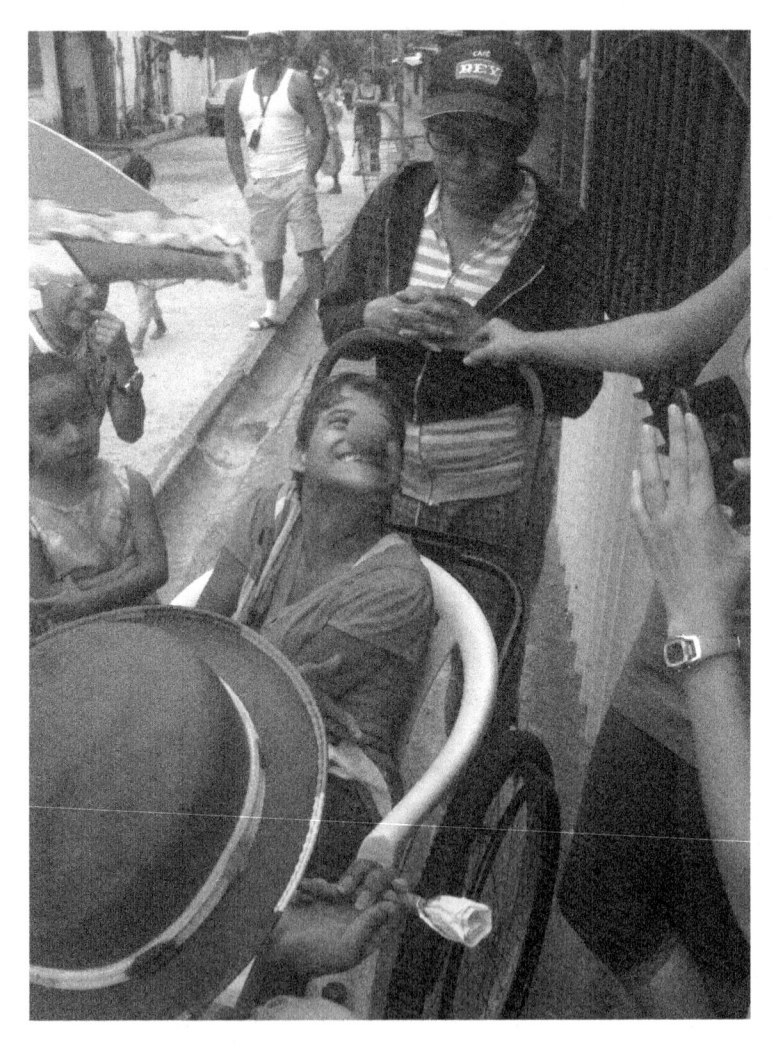

The residents had seen Patch and his clowns in Septembers past and looked forward to the special time when the clowns come. In the safety of daylight, the children of La Carpio came out to play with the clowns as the mothers cautiously looked on, appreciating us with returned smiles for the sunshine and joy we brought to their neighborhood. Parading in the streets and meeting each watchful eye with our own, connecting, understanding, sharing fun moments, a hug, a song, a dance, a paper flower. Small yet beautiful pearls emerged from the greatness of despair. We shared ourselves for just a short time, but the memory of it lasts a lifetime. Loving is the lesson Patch conveys to his clown groups. The powerful tool of human compassion delivered by the power of the red nose is the key.

"Clowning is a trick to bring love close," Patch teaches.

The memories of this day alone are as fresh today as they were then. When moments are as powerful as these, it becomes imprinted so vividly in your human experience. I still recall many scenes like this.

Back on our bus for the return trip to the hostel, there were quiet tears from exhausted clowns. La Carpio faded away behind us as images of many happy faces burned into our memories.

Good night, dear friends. We can play again tomorrow.

On our second day, we resumed our clowning tour, but this time in the rougher parts of La Carpio, near the river. With the experiences of a full day of street clowning already behind us, we were better prepared (so we thought) with fresh ideas that emerged following the culture shock and acclimation to the environment we experienced on the first day. We were a little more seasoned and more comfortable in our roles. We began to feel as though we had an invisible force field that encircled us. Within this clown bubble, no fear, danger, or violence dared to enter. This protection was necessary because we brought clowns to a much more primitive area that made the first neighborhoods seem like a modern suburb. We were swimming in the deep end of despair now for sure. Being a clown there was much harder, all the while your heart was breaking for the children and families living on the banks of a brown river, in huts made from scrap materials.

Frequently at our mission locations, the clown group would break up into smaller squads to cover more ground. We were always in earshot of accordion music played by Susan Parenti, longtime partner to Patch and founder of the School for Designing a Society. [7] Susan was a delightful leader in guiding our experiences and also rounded us up with her music when it came time to regroup. Herding clowns is a tough assignment, but there can be no clown left behind.

Later that afternoon, we followed the sounds of the accordion to head back to the "civilized" sections. We concluded our clowning rounds and gathered to pay a visit to a women's shelter located on the second floor of one of the few concrete structures in the "downtown" area on the main road into La Carpio. The shelter was on the second floor, accessible only by steep and narrow stairs.

Patch, at 67 years of age and wearing big floppy clown shoes, decided he would scoop Elizabeth out of her wheelchair and proceed up those stairs before anyone realized what he was doing. I was shocked that he did not ask for anyone's help and quickly followed up the stairs with the wheelchair so he could put her down once we got up there. Patch was impressed with Elizabeth and thrilled to have this courageous wheelchair-bound clown on the trip with him.

Once we settled into a large community room at the shelter, Patch and Eberhart, the ER doctor, stretched out Elizabeth's arms for some well-deserved relief of her spastic muscle tension. She was beaming, and we appreciated the concern Patch showed for her and all the needs of his clowns, both physical and emotional. We made Patch promise to allow us to do the heavy lifting on the trip back down the stairs when our visit at the women's shelter was over.

The women and children living in the shelter then presented a dramatic play they had prepared for our group to tell of their dangerous escape from Nicaragua to their newfound haven in La Carpio. After the show, they brought us into a small store room where we could buy handcrafted items to help support the shelter. We purchased a lot of stuff from these courageous ladies.

The next day after breakfast, we prepared for our next adventure. I looked forward to this day most of all because this was our first experience working with Patch in a hospital. We were going to meet up with the HospiSonrisas medical clowns at the National Children's Hospital in San Jose. [8] Patch had many friends there and it was a big deal when Gesundheit clowns came to visit. This annual clown reunion was a joy for all the staff, and many doctors and nurses came out to meet Patch.

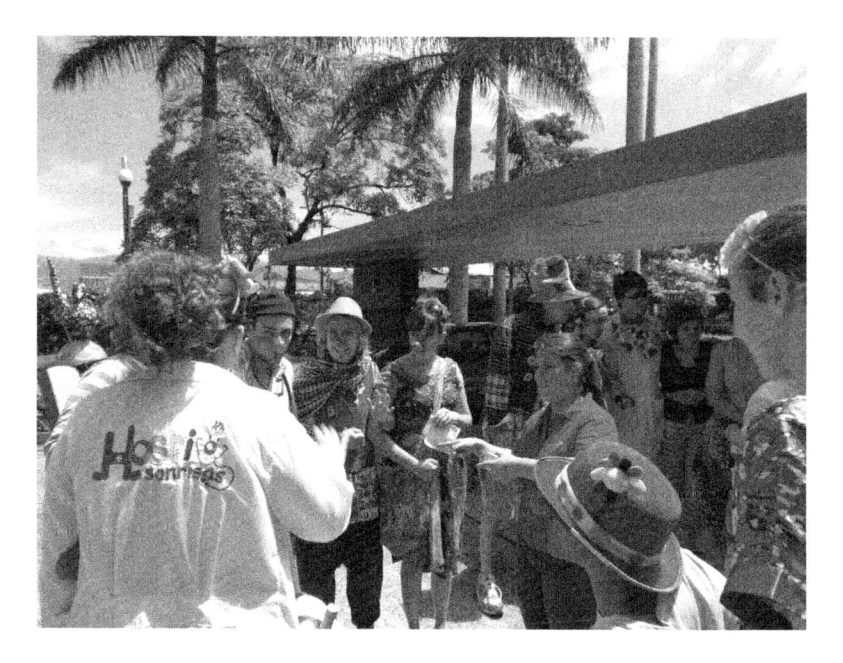

At the hospital, we met the medical clowns outside the front entrance. The hospital clowns were exquisite at sharing and guiding the experience for Patch's clowns as we broke off into our smaller groups to go to several different areas of the hospital. Dario brought Paloma, Gem, Elizabeth, Sadie, and myself to the burn unit. On the way, we were met with many joyful interactions in the hallways as the presence of clowns changed the reality for everyone we encountered. It was like walking through a sea of smiles and gratitude, and with each measured step, we became more energized in clown love. Getting your happy tank filled is pretty important because the energy empties quickly when you bring it into the darker places where pain and misery live.

In the burn unit, Antonio Zuniga Arbustini was a fantastic clown host. Not able to utter a single word in English and my dozen or so Spanish words not helping much, we communicated in pantomime and soon discovered we were carrying the same magic props. We instantly knew we had all we needed to put on a show together. Imagine one clown making a handkerchief disappear from one hand, then having it appear in the hand of the other clown across the room. Antonio had a magic red light at his fingertips too. We had a lovely game passing that magic light between us! All this was possible thanks to simple universal props magicians use. Antonio was a great clown partner, and our performance that day was sublime.

Paloma, Dario, Elizabeth, and Sadie each chose a child to interact with individually, and Antonio and I played to the larger room, trading off magic and other goofy shenanigans. Several of the children were motionless and quiet. Attended by family members, each child had a different threshold for pain and involvement with play was limited based on medical severity. The common playroom inside the burn unit was used to provide a safe space to escape from the daily routines of debridement, wound care, and other unpleasantness. Heavily medicated, though not fully finding relief, the children's eyes still followed the clowns with interest and curiosity, even if a smile was too hard to make.

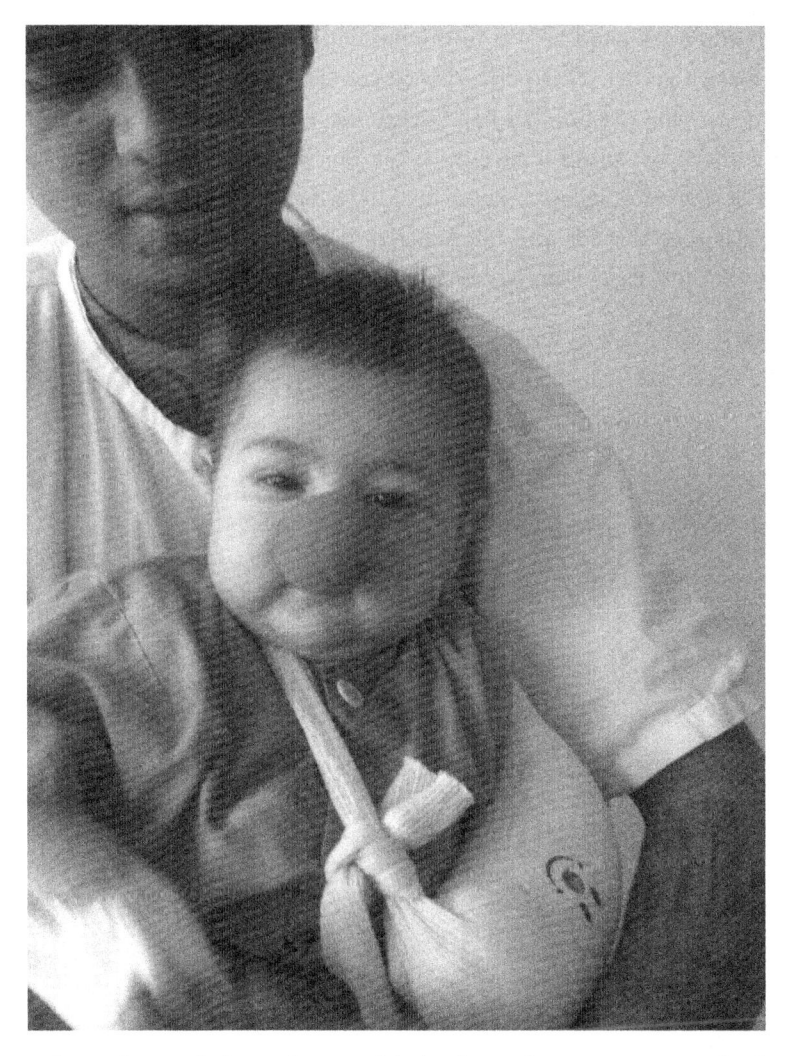

Antonio carried a guitar on his back, and soon we were singing songs. Paloma knew the words and sang beautifully. I did the best I could. We ended our show, said our happy goodbyes to the unit, and slowly worked our way through the halls, back to the front lobby, clowning with staff and patients all along the way.

Back outside we exchanged feedback with each other and members of the HospiSonrisas clowns. Dario translated for Antonio and me so we could talk about our experience. Dario told him I was also a pediatric nurse, and he was impressed with our ability to connect and perform together. This performance connection was where I credited my great clown school and the many magician mentors for the tools used that day. Antonio gave me a big hug and a pair of pink electric guitar shaped sunglasses from his clown bag as a gift to remember our day together. He and I connected that day, and thanks to Google translate and Facebook, we are still friends today!

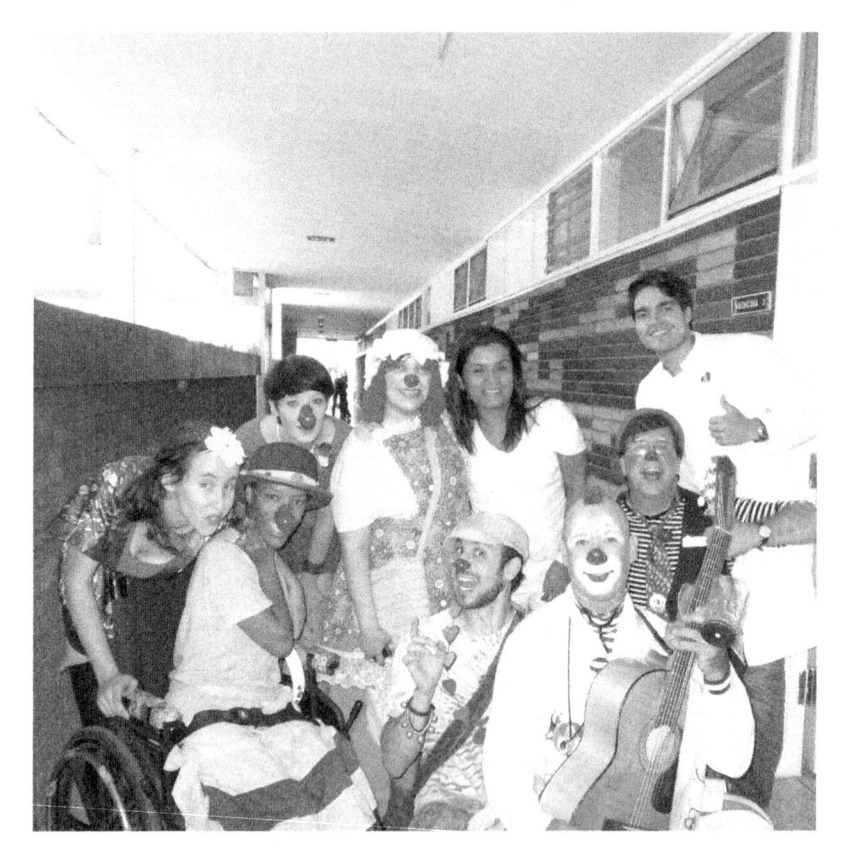

Patch and the Gesundheit staff provided many learning experiences during that week-long adventure. We shared meals together, stories, lectures, workshops, and group discussions each day, in addition to our clown outings. We bonded as a family. Patch had much to teach us about Love Strategy, a lesson in therapeutic touch and therapeutic communication. We learned how to be totally present for another person and connect with them, giving full focused attention. Jacob Barton, one of Patch's clown leaders, gave a powerfully moving lecture called "Making Big Things Small and Small Things Big." This presentation made us aware of how small actions of loving intent can overshadow a larger desperate condition, providing relief, even if only briefly, in the lives of others. This concept became clearer to us during our clown rounds each day. The 2012 Clowning and Caring mission had been very rewarding so far. I wondered what it would be like to do this work full time. What a great job that would be!

On the fourth day, the clown team ventured into the only mental hospital in Costa Rica. It was a large facility that housed patients young and old, separated by gender, wearing blue and pink scrub-like pajamas. There were multiple dormitory-like structures and open air lawns where most of the patients were free to move around on the grounds while loosely supervised by staff wearing white. The color scheme was easy to follow. We were the colorful ones, and easy to spot if trouble erupted.

I was walking along a covered path with Patch and a few other doctor and nurse clowns as we headed to the women's section when from several hundred yards away, we saw a screaming woman charging at full speed toward our clown group.

"Papeeee! Papeeee," she cried as she ran, carrying a baby doll under one arm. Her oversized pink pajamas were barely hanging on to her large undulating body as she zeroed in on us.

I thought Dr. Adams was about to get tackled when at the very last second, she wrapped herself around my stunned nurse friend Herb. They fell to the ground in a tangled mess as she bear-hugged her petrified clown. Herb's priceless expression of surprise was epic. We were quite amused watching Herb try in vain to peel her off. That clown was her Pappy, and she was obviously very glad he came to visit!

Patch spoke of his personal experiences with depression and being a patient himself in mental health facilities when he was younger. With his small group of medical clowns, Patch had great discussions about the state of healthcare in our country and the lack of proper mental health care.

"I never disliked anyone enough to prescribe a psychotropic medication," Patch said with impunity.

He told us about a time when he hugged a schizophrenic patient for several hours during a psychotic break just to keep him safe and connected to another human being. He shared his feelings on euthanasia, and how we are so ready to ease suffering for our beloved pets, but it is never an option for human suffering.

"No one will ever visit these people here," he said. "Would you like to have the option of choosing a humane end to your suffering if you could?"

We spent an hour or so working with the women in pink out on the lawn. We each found an opportunity to play with the patients in fascinating and unique ways. Language barriers and lack of sanity presented no difficulty for creative clowning. Music and juggling scarves played well for me.

I noticed one woman restrained in a wheelchair, her wrists tightly bound to the arms of her chair with sheets. She was parked well away from the other patients, alone. I presumed it was either as punishment or she just didn't play well with others. I was drawn to her specifically, wanting to check her circulation and restraints to make sure they were not too tight. I pushed two fingers into the snug loops around her wrists and brought some slight relief for her. It was a little tight.

The lady appeared to be in her forties, sad and slow to react. I couldn't tell if she was restrained to prevent self-harm or harm to others, but decided I would try to interact with her. I brought out my colored juggling scarves, placed one in each of my hands, and sang a little melody as I waved them back and forth. I then put them into her hands, and she took them from me with a pinching movement of her fingers, clearly understanding the game was about gripping and releasing the scarves. I began to move the scarves between her two hands and my own, and she gripped and released accordingly. Soon we were juggling three scarves together, passing them from hand to hand. As we played together, I relished in the thought that as the mental health workers in white watched on, I helped one of the inmates escape from her isolation even if just a little bit, for a little while, her hands bound but face smiling as we juggled those scarves. It was a glorious moment. She had a playmate that day, but how many other days had she been parked away from the group to sit alone?

Juggling with this poor woman whose hands were tied, I found power through this new clown game. I felt very good about this simple, non-verbal connection.

In this section of the grounds, there were about 30 to 40 women spread around in smaller groups, so I continued on to find more to do. Making my way among groups of patients, I found another lady who looked at me with curiosity and smiled. I saw this as an invitation to visit, so I went to her to play. I tried the singing-juggling bit again just as before, and she responded favorably, looking quite enthusiastically at the colored scarves. I taught her the juggling game where we passed them to each other, but she had other plans. Passing the pink and blue scarves went well, but once she had the yellow scarf in her grasp, she ran away with it.

Uh oh, new game, I thought, and began the chase to recover the scarf. With only one set of juggling scarves in my possession, I had to negotiate a favorable resolution to this unexpected situation.

She never broke into a full run, but maintained a very intentional fast walk, designed to shake me from her tail. She weaved in and out around the groups of women seated on the lawn, frequently glancing back at me to see if I was still behind her. During this entire chase scene, I could not help but hear the Benny Hill theme song in my head as it played to the scenario perfectly. I used my best funny clown walk, of course. Several times we stopped and faced each other, and I would make a pleading gesture for the return of the scarf, extending my upturned hat and pointing to encourage her to deposit the stolen goods inside. She did not reconsider her position easily, and we continued our serpentine dance around the ladies in the yard.

"Persistence overcomes resistance," I had always said, and eventually we faced off for the last time.

Breathing heavily and glistening with perspiration from our funny little chase scene, she placed the scarf in my hat with an apologetic look. Suddenly taking a posture and expression of what appeared to me as guilt and remorse, she surprised me with yet another unexpected turn. She threw her body backward to the ground, landing with a thud in what I imagined was an action of self-punishment. She put herself in time out.

As I looked at her lying on the ground, I could not allow her to take total blame for the theft. After all, I did encourage her to play scarves with me. So I decided in the act of solidarity to follow her lead and throw myself backward to the ground too. We were both resting comfortably on the ground, staring up at a deep blue sky with puffy white clouds.

We laid on the ground next to each other for a very long time. Personally, I was grateful for the time to catch my breath. I glanced over to see how she was doing a few times. She looked pretty content and may have also needed the rest. I just relaxed and stared up into the sky, making a full assessment of my current condition.

I realized that I was fulfilling a dream I had not fully understood until that moment. There I was, lying on the ground next to a patient in a state-run psychiatric facility in Costa Rica, peacefully contemplating the deeper meanings of where I was in time and space. I felt my breathing ease as the grass from the lawn massaged my neck. I appreciated the shapes of the clouds framed in blue while taking in the fullness of the moment—I was on a mission trip with the real Patch Adams, and each extraordinary experience I had was changing me, broadening my humanity. I could see more clearly what my personal mission was becoming. I was a clown and a nurse, and all my gifts were meant to be healing. I wondered if it mattered whether my mother knew or not that I would find myself in this condition because of a wish she inspired.

I knew then that I was solely responsible for the life I was living. I was a clown—a real clown. I felt peace in my soul upon truly understanding what I went there to do.

*Clown is a verb more than a noun. It is
an action more than a character.*

Clowning was indeed a trick to bring love close, for yourself first and most importantly. Only then will you be properly equipped to love others when it is needed most. This realization was an epiphany moment, a real psychological breakthrough for me, and I would never have imagined it would arrive in this manner, in this very unusual place.

Rested and filled with gratitude for the experiences this September morning brought, I looked over at my playmate. When our eyes met again, I sat up and thanked her for sharing her time with me. I pulled out a colored napkin from my vest and began to make a gift for my friend. She sat up too and watched carefully at what I was doing. As I twisted the paper napkin into a rose, she recognized halfway through what it was becoming and was happy again. I gave her a yellow flower, and she accepted it gladly. All was right in our world again.

The clown team later assembled in the children's section of the campus, in a large open room with an adjacent walled courtyard along one side of the building. With boys in blue and girls in pink, we became the clown chaperones to what felt like a school dance and a pajama party combined. We were accompanied by some helpful counselors who assisted with our interactions, sharing with us the diagnosis and typical behaviors of the children. Some patients had schizophrenia, some were autistic, others had been molested or raped leaving them with severe anxiety and depression. The ages were mostly between 10 to 16 and evenly mixed of boys and girls.

Our clown team moved about the playroom, engaging small

groups of kids. I made good use of my close-up magic effects as this was the ideal age range. I was with a small semicircle of kids for what seemed a very long time and used all the magic props I had with me. Because of the clown gags I learned at New York Goof School, I never lacked for additional material. A clown's hat alone is a sacred prop full of comic possibilities. My distressed black top hat became a highly-prized commodity with the kids too. It found its way around the room on children's heads as they strolled around in newfound characters, displaying themselves joyfully to each other. The hat game was a common one among several other kids and clowns, so many other clown hats floated around that day too. They wanted us to take their pictures in our hats with our camera phones so they could see themselves. I then realized that the children were playing dress up and the hats added a much-needed fashion accessory to the drab blue and pink scrubs they wore every day of their confined lives. For those precious moments, they found new identities with our hats. I wondered how much these kids hated those scrubs.

After a long while, we all felt that our schoolyard recess was well spent. There was a sense of joy and satisfaction among all the clowns. Sharing this experience and watching Patch work his magic with these children will stay with me forever. Words cannot adequately describe the impact this day had on me. The connections we made with the patients were rich with valuable lessons in our basic humanity. The power of clowning as a method for relief work was clearly evident in this place. I had never been more thankful to be a caregiver.

The last destination of our clown adventure brought the team to the state prison on the fifth and final mission day. The fun began when we arrived and learned we would be carefully screened and possibly strip searched by armed guards before being allowed through the first gate. I thought the TSA agents were bad; these guys had guns and were very skilled at patting you down. I endured the intimate moment with light humor and was relieved no cavity search was necessary. There is only so much I was willing to suffer for my art. I still needed a cigarette afterward, though.

Each experience of clowning in La Carpio, the children's hospital, and the psychiatric institute demonstrated the challenges of distressed people under different circumstances. The common thread was that "bad" came in many forms, but humanity was also present in each place and could be nourished by the clown, no matter what the harsh circumstance. The prison would show us the hardened reality of violence, isolation, and despair on a new level.

The state prison housed adult and children prisoners. We were led to a large common room under guard, where we were to have visitation with the juvenile inmates. They were seated in plastic chairs on the perimeter, against all four walls, and had angry, stone-like expressions on their faces as they sat with defensive postures. Girls on one side, boys on the other. Guards strategically posted themselves around the room. We sensed instantly that this was going to be a tough sell. I recalled one of the guards had shared with us that some of these kids would say they are in for murder just to ward off harassment from other kids. Some did commit murder. Hard to tell the difference from our perspective.

With such hardened glares surrounding us clowns all bunched together in the center, we broke our huddle, selected our targets, and expanded out to fill the space. Reluctant at first, the faces on the kids began to relax and arms started to uncross. I started with my close-up magic routines, which began pulling them out of chairs into a half circle to watch my wizardry. About fifteen minutes into the action, the entire room looked more like any middle school gym (except for the guards) as we were all now moving about and playing together.

The kids were hesitant to melt at first because no one wanted to let down their guard, but as clowns, we penetrated their tough exteriors and invited ridicule on ourselves first. Then it became the game, and all the defenses came down.

After a fun filled hour of playing, our time was coming to an end. Melanie, our Gesundheit guide, suggested we wrap up our show by performing Clown Machine. This routine was an improvisation exercise where a single clown begins by taking a position on stage and making a movement and a sound of some kind. Each subsequent clown adds to the scene with a new sound and motion, and this continues on until all clowns are crammed together, each doing their thing, building the clown machine. This colorful moving mass of noisy clown sculpture was a spectacle and allowed for passive observation as the kids found their chairs again.

Slowly the mood began to change, and the children's expressions lost that brief burst of innocence to resume those stoic prison faces again. Only they wore smiley stickers on their shirts, which I passed out like prison cigarettes. This image seemed surreal to me.

Once we finished our last game, the children were told to return to the seats around the perimeter as we remained in the center. The guards walked around the room to place handcuffs on all the kids and counted them. Then they were made to line up to be attached to long metal chains for the return to their confinement quarters.

We could see a look of shame mixed with gratitude on some of those faces, and a few others with hardened faces made eye contact and gave a little nod of the head. They were glad we came.

The prison kids were shackled together in tight rows. We could see their reality more clearly than when we arrived. Those initial prison faces returned as the guards marched them quietly back to their cells.

Back on the bus with the memories of this final day added to the previous ones, we collectively felt satisfaction mixed with sadness just as we had at the end of each adventure. Patch shared more of his experiences from past trips as we debriefed from that mission outing.

Patch Adams had long hair worn in a ponytail that was blue on one side, gray on the other, and he wore a small fork as an earring. He told us the fork was a reminder that children are dying every day for lack of food. He'd held several children in his arms who would die only days later of starvation. His colorful clothing was always easily and instantly transformed into his clown persona whenever he wanted. He showed us in his example how easy it was to keep your clown power close at hand for whenever it was needed. It's not hard to see that as a physician, there really is no one else quite like Patch. I can't say I have ever met anyone else who exceeded his brilliance, intellect, energy, and compassion. Though he does not prescribe to any particular faith, he embraces people of all faiths throughout the world and has prayed with anyone who desired it, because it was an act of love for the other person. Love and friendship are truly his greatest gifts to a hurting world!

Learning how to be a humanitarian clown can change a person. The power behind the clown's ability to "make big things small and small things big" as Jacob Barton showed us, and "bringing love close," the principle Patch taught, was demonstrated to us over and again with each day's field work. We learned how to relieve a person's mind from anxiety and redirect their experience momentarily through the compassionate work of humanitarian clowning. Simply by bringing ourselves to focused attention, being present and genuinely loving, we discovered how the red nose invited access to another person's suffering to relieve them. Each evening we dined together as a family and told stories to each other deep into the night.

You never forget your first clown troupe or your first season as a "First of May" clown.

A medical emergency at home had me flying out a day early, and Patch too had to return to the US the following day. The clown team spent their final day free to roam, rest, and explore Costa Rica.

Many people go to Costa Rica for the beaches, resorts, great vacations. We went to explore the dark places and bring a little light and love. We each were searching for something inside ourselves, to learn what wisdom the good clown doctor could teach us. Dr. Adams is a great physician whose life and work is still changing the world through the expanding wake of friends he makes.

Soon after my return to Texas, I was on fire to find clowning opportunities to serve in my community. I volunteered Tater to numerous special events and put into practice what I had learned. Making hospital clown visits and entertaining for medical causes I supported helped me find more ways to integrate creativity into my regular nursing practice too.

In one of our evening conversations, Patch had told me I should try to find a way to help other nurses fight stress and burn out like I had done using magic. I was both mad scientist and guinea pig as I learned how to combine magic and clown arts with nursing. It would take some divine assistance to pull this all together, and I pray for more opportunities for this work to grow.

This is the magic nurse mission, and I hope you will jump in the noodles with me!

CHAPTER 7

HOSPITAL MAGIC

*"The art of medicine consists of keeping the
patient amused while nature heals the disease."*

—*Voltaire*

MAGIC NURSE, LLC WAS ORGANIZED as a sole proprietor corporation in February 2012. My mission was to provide the right kind of creative, therapeutic entertainment that would be to the best benefit of patients and their families at the exact right time. I provide hospital visits for bedside performances as a clinical entertainer. Each hospital visit arranged with thoughtful planning by close family is a custom show. As a nurse, I am familiar with the clinical environment, changing conditions, need for rest, and timing of treatments. Coordinating with each family is necessary to ensure that we plan a beneficial experience for the patient.

Often the patient is told a special visitor is coming. Sometimes the family wants a surprise visit by the silly clown doctor. Either way, I am not like any other hospital visitor they have ever seen before. I bring a musical, magical comedy performance to the bedside where we all play together. Teleporting ourselves for the moment into a world of imagination, I bring a variety of props to tailor whatever feels right at the moment. Everyone in the room takes part in the creation of the experience. I am a facilitator for helping patients and families release their joy. Clearly, this is the best use of art I have ever experienced, and I cannot imagine a better reason for doing it. I am a professional visitor and friend with the capability to entertain and be an advocate for a healing experience. I share magic with them, and they get a nurse friend for free.

It was obvious I couldn't pull my little clown car up to any hospital and start seeing patients, so I had to create a pathway into the clinical environment. I needed the ability to visit anyone, anywhere, at any time to do my thing. To accomplish this creative clinical work, I needed access by invitation as a requested hospital visitor. The best way possible, I discovered, was to become a professional visitor, the same as any visiting priest or pastor. I operate as a nurse/clown/magician with a performance art ministry.

Needing a way for people to find me, I had to advertise my services. I had to think of a way to share the concept of what I did to the public in a way that made sense to them. So I looked at the traditional way friends and relatives cheer patients up:

They send flowers.

I packaged my service visit to be a gift you could send that was cheaper than flowers. For a small fee, you could arrange a magic nurse visit for anyone at any hospital. I also made emergency visits for parents of a child with an urgent need at no cost. The price of dialing their phone was all I needed, and I would find a way to get there. Making house calls and hospital visits whenever it was needed is the purpose of this mission. The transaction was only a way to get the wheels in motion.

My advertisement suggested an alternative to traditional get well gifts. My goal was not to profit from the visit, but to gain access to the clinical spaces. As an invited guest to the patient's bedside, I have the privilege of sharing my healing art in a needed situation for families and patients.

I get many requests from friends, colleagues, and other associates. Once I got a call from a talent agent who got a desperate call from a single mother. Her son was in the hospital on his birthday. The agent knew I was the one for the job, and I visited them within hours of her call at no charge. My business was to make these visits whenever and wherever they were needed, but I did not want any family to pay for my work. They'd already paid a high price, and my purpose was not just to help them, but anyone else I found that needed comic relief along the way.

The scope of my service is more than just seeing scheduled patients. The invitation to the bedside was only one part of the plan, the first point of entry into the hospital system. Once inside the clinical space, I was now available to entertain anyone I had the chance to meet. This opportunity is the gift I had in mind to deliver performance art into any hospital I happened to visit.

You can imagine stealth is impossible when you are in costume. It is evident a clown has arrived at the scene, and I am in character as soon as I am visible. I appear as a silly looking clown doctor, and even though clown shoes are sticking out from under the lab coat, my proper clown behavior is somewhat reserved. As I walk into the hospital, I engage every smiling face I meet with a return smile and tip of the hat, and my work has begun.

I am there to brighten the environment with my presence on the way in and on the way out because it is a natural side effect and benefit of my arrival to see my patient. I do not hurry; I'm not limited by time. I take a natural pace and benefit from any opportunity to share with someone who engages me. I am anyone's clown who needs it. Each of these random encounters is just as important as the scheduled one.

Once I make it to the medical floor of my patient, I check in with the nurse's station to inform them of the purpose of my visit and which specific patient I have been requested to see. I tell them I am a registered nurse also and ask if there are any special precautions or treatments in progress I should be aware of before entering the room. I frequently get an inquisitive look as they are processing the odd combination of nurse and clown. These introductions are great because they give me a chance to share with very surprised nurses how and why I do this work. I get many opportunities to share my mission and show them magic tricks also. They don't know it, but I came to share with them too. They benefit from a pleasant diversion and get a glimpse into a creative way they too can express care to patients. It is like planting a seed for a potential future where more of this kind of work may grow.

"This could be you after twenty years of nursing!" I say, and that is always good for a laugh.

But I am serious.

I always make time to see as many other patients as possible. I usually ask the nurses if they have someone special they would like me to see. After visiting my first patient, often there are several more lined up for me when I return to the desk.

The nurses also benefit from the funny distraction from their daily routines. A moment of abandon and unexpected humor that arrives unannounced makes the surprise that much more pleasant. Like a magic trick has that instant moment of surprise, so does the appearance of a clown doctor on the unit. Stressful conditions in a hospital can affect everyone, most especially nurses. The demands of modern nursing have increased exponentially with new technologies, higher acuity of patients, and increasing patient assignments. Having a brief moment of intellectual relief by an unexpected clown can make for a lasting effect on mood and attitude.

I call this "ambush clowning," and as the term suggests, the element of surprise is to my advantage. The stress relief is instant and efficient. Sharing magic, music, paper roses, and red noses with the staff is just as rewarding for me because providing a moment of joyful distraction from their crappy day while showing them a possibility they can consider for their practice too is at the heart of my mission. I give away clown noses and for a moment, we all become nurse clowns. They get a glimpse into my world, and once the noses are on, the camera phones come out to capture this funny moment. We are creating a message and sending it out to the universe to say we desire better for ourselves and our patients. We need to laugh more!

I carry a ukulele strapped on my back and a doctor bag full of magic. I come to play for as long as I am needed. Nursing assessment skills, behind the red nose, allow me to recognize the subtle clues nurses quickly detect to gauge their patient for the actions best suited for the moment. I know when to shift into another gag or effect, or what song to play to make the time sweet, loving, fun, and beautiful for the family. More especially, I know when to end the show and exit with grace.

This is the pinnacle of performing art for me. The feedback is immediate and the experience unique every time. Sometimes just sitting with them and letting them share their experiences with me becomes the game. Listening is important for both adult and child patients. I have the time and patience to be a supportive ear, and I am an understanding medical professional/clown who is totally present and available for them.

To further the therapeutic value magic has, patients can also learn selected magic tricks that support their healing. I have some favorite magic tricks I teach patients who desire to learn them, and I give them props to keep so they can practice and perform their magic tricks for others.

Napkin roses are another favorite item I use. I make a performance out of the first one, then hold a mini class for the patient and family to make some of their own. The power of giving something like a magic trick to practice or a stack of colored napkins to make roses leaves a lasting impression of my visit of course, but more importantly, it gives the patient a new activity, a new focus they did not have before. Napkin roses are both a great memento and simple skill to acquire, providing enjoyment long after I have gone.

When the patient encounter is over, I make my way back to the nurses' station where the remainder of my adventure can unfold into many different directions. I often meet a nurse manager or charge nurse and have the opportunity to share my mission. The curiosity of where I came from and how I came about doing this work is a great conversation, and I make new nurse friends everywhere I go. It helps that I am a clinical nurse and my credentials are easily verifiable. I am often guided to visit other patients and families. Word travels fast when a clown shows up on the unit, and many new invitations generate once I arrive. I always plan to stay a while because that was the goal all along.

I walk out of the hospital the same way I meandered in, making the most out of chance encounters along the way. Each hospital I visit adds to the collection of meaningful experiences that continue to shape my understanding of the social value of this clinical clown work.

Magic Nurse has been a passion for me from the very first time I saw how a simple magic trick made a difference in a young patient's life. As I repeated this experiment, I found positive outcomes each time. Becoming a clown opened my eyes to the healing value of all the creative arts. I had to see how far it could go.

I'm still going!

CHAPTER 8
BRETT'S STORY

"Never leave a friend behind. Friends are all we have to get us through this life—and they are the only things from this world that we could hope to see in the next."

—Dean Koontz, Fear Nothing

I HAD A VERY CLOSE FRIEND who relocated to Heaven just two years prior to writing this book, and there is not a day I don't think of him at least once. Neither one of us could have imagined how our friendship would take the fateful turns we experienced together. The impact Brett had on me solidified how necessary my clinical magic and clown work would become. Brett was my mentor, and I loved him like a brother. He helped define for me what it meant to be a "magic nurse." Performing both as a clinical partner and creative friend. The artist at the bedside.

For magicians, friendships carry an extra connection because we don't separate the magic from the magician who created it. For every magic routine and many props and card sleights, the credit for it goes to the magician who first developed it. We honor their memory by connecting their name forever to their unique contribution to the art. Elmsley's count, Goshman's pinch, or Down's palm are just a few examples of this tradition keeping these men alive forever in the hands of future generations of magicians.

Brett Wolf may not have his name attached to a card maneuver or any piece of magic in particular, but his magic is embedded deeply in the hearts of too many magicians to list. I am just one of them; the last one, sadly. Brett was an amazingly talented magician blessed with such generosity and compassion to help others. His most appreciated gift was the ability to recognize the possibilities in anyone's performance. He taught me much during our time together and had done so much more for many others in the years before we met.

Brett was a true friend to many top magicians and the kind of guy who had a genuine warmth with people and made friends easily. He was barely forty years old when he died, though he had accomplished a lot of magic during his life. I could not possibly write adequate words to honor his life or his memory. This chapter is not the whole story of Brett, but just that small piece of time he shared with me. I owe an enormous debt of gratitude for his help with MagicNurse.com. Our chance meeting and the times to follow would put everything I had learned in both art and medicine to the test.

I met Brett and his fiancé Robyn in October 2012, very soon after my trip to Costa Rica with Patch. We met while volunteering for a Make-A-Wish train ride event on a special BNSF luxury passenger train that took a 3-hour trip filled with special kids and their families. Leaving from the historic Stockyard Station in Ft. Worth, the train was well staffed with an army of volunteer entertainers, magicians, clowns, musicians, face painters, and balloon artists.

I was Tater that day and volunteered with my clown friend Hattie. She and I were thrilled to spend the day clowning for the kids. I spent the time performing magic for small groups of children, moving from car to car. A couple of hours into the ride, I stepped into the lounge car to rehydrate and, as I was savoring my bottled water, a fellow who had watched me perform struck up a conversation.

"I noticed you were doing magic over there." He smiled.

"Yea, I just do simple tricks, nothing fancy," I said. "I keep my magic easy, tricks found in magic sets for kids eight and up."

"That's great, though. That's when most magicians get started," he said.

"Are you a magician?" I asked.

"Yes, I am actually. I'm new to Dallas, though."

I then proceeded to tell him about the Dallas Magic Club and the great lecture series of top professional magicians that come through. I was especially excited to tell him about the next magic lecture coming up the following week.

"He's a great pro magician. Brett Wolf's his name, and he worked with David Copperfield, The Amazing Kreskin, Bill Malone," I said. "He's supposed to be really good."

"I believe I am actually going to that lecture," he said. "I'm Brett Wolf."

Yes, I'm an idiot. Not surprising at all that a random clown on a train would invite a master magician to his own lecture. We joked a lot about this later. This funny little Tater moment guaranteed I was not going to miss that lecture.

Brett introduced me to his lovely Robyn, and our friendship grew that day and in the weeks afterward. With the Patch Adams adventure still fresh in my head, I shared the stories of my Costa Rica experiences with Brett. He was very interested in learning more about Patch and had some ideas he felt could help him in his quest to raise more money for his institute. Brett called Copperfield, who arranged a call with Patch to make an introduction.

Patch and Brett spoke several times, and Brett shared his ideas for a touring project. Managing touring shows was one of Brett's many talents. He'd just finished a road tour for Rain, a Beatles Tribute band. Patch was interested in exploring this idea. Meanwhile, Robyn was about to open a retail store called Ra Ra's Closet in the Lake Highlands area in Dallas. The grand opening was happening on Saturday, December 8th, 2012, and Brett asked if I would mind performing for the event. Brett expressed a keen interest in what I was trying to accomplish with Magic Nurse and put his mind to finding ways to help me. I could not have been more grateful for Brett's assistance and was very happy to help with Robyn's grand opening.

Brett had excellent graphic art skills and wanted to help me develop my brand. It is hard to describe exactly what a "Magic Nurse" is and why anyone would need one. There certainly is value to caring for people with magic and art, but not typically a good return on investment for business. He embraced the challenge I was facing in doing the work I desired most while finding a way to support it financially.

He went to work on my mission and created an advertisement promoting my website MagicNurse.com, which he was going to run in a local children's magazine. Robyn also used this publication for her retail advertising, and they knew the publisher personally. When the editor heard about what I was doing, he did not charge for the ad and ran it monthly for free! I could not have been more grateful for this because I was covering costs of my magic adventures with my regular nursing job and clown gigs.

I had not actually charged anyone for a hospital visit yet and never intended to profit from the patients. I hoped to find supporters or outside contacts wishing to hire me as a gift rather than sending flowers. Magic Nurse, LLC was a clinical entertainment business with no financial plan or hope of making a profit. I volunteered a lot and kept my regular nursing job to cover my business. I marketed Tater for birthdays and events for a while, and that helped too. Ultimately, I knew I should try to become a nonprofit, but for now, I just wanted to see more patients.

On the Grand Opening of Ra Ra's Closet, Tater the Clown spent a great day with friends and tons of kids and families. Robyn and Brett had worked hard to get the store ready, and opening day was a blast. While we were hanging out after closing time, catching our breath and having Migas from J.J.'s café next door, Brett told me that if he were ever to be a clown, he thought Sucker Punch the Clown would be a great name. We laughed about it, but he could not have suspected how it would come back to bite him. A terrible blow was about to be delivered. We never saw it coming.

It was just a week later when I received a desperate call from Robyn telling me Brett was in the ICU at St. Paul Medical Center in critical condition. The panic in her voice and the weight of her words were devastating. She said he was taken by ambulance to St. Paul ER and needed emergency surgery for acute internal bleeding. A second surgery to stop the bleeding was necessary only a couple of hours following the first, and multiple blood transfusions were given to keep him stable. The large volume blood loss was very bad by itself, but with the additional news of severe liver damage and toxic ammonia levels, the situation was critical if not dire.

"I need a clown up here, Rob! Brett needs a clown!"

They both needed a friend, and she needed hope. This plea may have sounded like an odd request to most people, but I knew what it meant. She needed a large dose of clown love and positive energy to claim victory over this event and help her believe Brett was going to come out of this okay.

"I'm on my way, Robyn, but I'm bringing clown noses for all of us."

I was still in my scrubs from work, but I grabbed my clown doctor hat, lab coat, doctor bag full of magic, and off I went. I brought a couple of new clown noses I had ordered special from a theatrical mask maker out of Chicago—Jeff Semmerling, who also makes clown noses for the staff at Gesundheit Institute. These noses had a new special purpose; they were going to be used to help my friends.

When I arrived at the hospital, Robyn met me in the parking lot to fill me in on details and take me up to the ICU. Brett's mother Karen had just flown in from her home in Ohio and was at his bedside, keeping watch. It was right then and there, in that dark parking lot that I initiated Robyn into medical clowning, Patch Adams style.

"You put on a nose. You're a clown!" Patch declares.

It's that simple.

I placed one of the Semmerling noses on Robyn and declared her a clown. It was a simple battlefield promotion. I told Robyn just to be aware of the looks people give you when they make eye contact. If they smile, they are inviting you; just smile back and share your joy with them like you would anyone else you would meet in passing, just a little happier than normal.

"Let that random meeting be whatever it becomes for them, and just love them!" I said. "Just be the most joyful expression of yourself and keep it honest."

As we walked into the hospital, we clowned for everyone we passed by on the way. With her clown nose, pink juggling scarf tied in her hair, and my oversized lab coat hanging from her, Robyn found the power of the red nose very quickly. She had a natural love for people, and we were getting warmed up for the ICU.

When we reached the ICU floor, Robyn hit the big silver button opening the double doors into the unit, and we arrived on the scene to deliver fearless clown energy to every person who needed it, beginning with Brett.

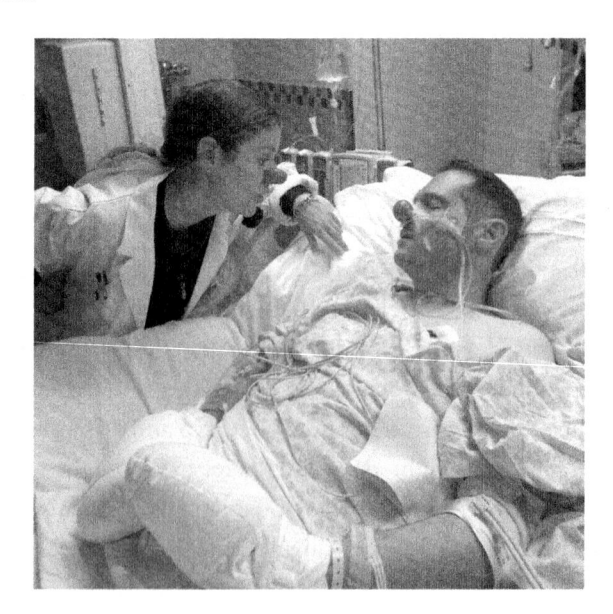

At first glance, I noticed they had Brett in soft wrist restraints that looked like big white boxing mitts. Tubes entered and exited all the usual places you would expect on a critical patient. Robyn told me he was delirious, combative, and restless following surgery as he drifted in and out of consciousness. Restraints were used to prevent pulling out tubes and IVs in this altered state. He must have unknowingly exercised some of his escape artist talents after surgery.

"Sucker Punch!" I exclaimed at the sight of him "You still have your boxing gloves on!"

I then noticed his mother Karen standing in the corner.

"Oh, hi. It's okay, I'm a medical professional," I said.

"Hey, I brought your nose!" turning back to Brett.

I placed the second Semmerling nose on Brett, and we could see him starting to stir a bit. Robyn and I talked to him and clowned with him as his world came in and out of focus. I visited with Karen also and shared with her how Brett and I met, and about how he helped with my clinical magic and clowning work. I let her in on our "Sucker Punch" joke, and she appreciated the cliff notes on our clown connection. The red noses planted on Brett and Robyn's faces gave me the sense that we were ready for anything. Robyn then encouraged me to visit some of the other patients she had met, and off we went on clown rounds to see everyone in the intensive care unit at Saint Paul Medical Center.

Wherever we met friendly and inviting eyes, we asked permission to play. We made paper napkin roses to share, played music, did magic and gave away clown noses and smiley stickers to anyone who wanted to play with us. We loved them with our art and connected as friends, silly and funny clown friends. Robyn was a natural clown, letting her friendly presence fill each room with kindness. In return, the sincere appreciation and smiles we experienced from these men and women were warm and gracious. The nursing staff had never seen anything like us on their unit before. Clowns are for kids, right? We found that nurses and doctors were ready to play too. I shared my magic nurse story and showed them magic tricks I used in the clinical setting. Nurses needed to know what I had discovered, and I shared the story of my clinical magic journey wherever I could find a willing ear and interest.

After about an hour of visiting the ICU neighbors, we returned to Brett's room to encourage him further. This time he started waking up and was able to focus on us in brief intervals. His nurse was a sweet young lady who had no problem putting on one of the sponge clown noses also. It happened to be her birthday that day. Brett was good enough now to have his mitts removed, and his hands were free to touch things. He was drowsy but now talking with us, making sure all the while his nose was on straight.

Was this a miracle? I cannot say, but it was a very good turn of events to be sure. Brett would later recall after leaving the hospital several days later that this was his only memory of this first hospitalization. Two nurses, his fiancé, and most of the adults in Brett's room wearing clown noses. I'm sure his mom Karen, who flew in from Ohio to see her son, now had a very strange and memorable impression of Texans.

This sudden immersion in adult medical clowning was surprisingly an easy transition from working with kids. I felt a stronger desire to find relief for a moment from the inviting looks in their eyes as they motioned me in from the doorway. We approached gently in each case, being mindful of whoever was in the room and finding acceptance to share a few moments with them. We offered sponge clown noses to anyone who wished to play with us, and that small act alone often brought new energy for everyone present. I made napkin roses for the patients to give as a token of love to their husbands and wives, a small act of empowerment to let the patient show a bit of love and give a little gift to their partners.

Adults were a lot easier to clown for because they clearly know the clown is not just there for silliness but to offer them a distraction, playful relief, and a few moments of joyful peace. In the wake of the smiley stickers we placed on patient hospital gowns and medical scrubs of doctors and nurses, we marked a trail of love energy and appreciated the impact, and the lives we touched by merely being present in that unit. Boldly leading with our Clown Power and humbling ourselves to become compassionate fools.

Brett left the hospital stable and recovering a few days later, but faced some new challenges. His liver was badly damaged, and he would have to be very careful with diet and lifestyle. He was closely monitored by his doctors and eventually going to need a liver transplant. Brett and Robyn were a strong team, and with her extensive knowledge of nutrition and his incredible intellect, they took every step necessary to bring healing to his body in the following months. He gained strength and seemed to be getting better. The next six months would show continued promise for improvement.

Brett and I visited often and had magic sessions whenever we could. Being active in other magic circles, we often ran into each other at Magic venues and other meeting groups. Brett had a keen interest in my Magic Nurse work; he was fascinated at how I approached clowning from a medical aspect and the psychology involved in finding the right trick or clown moment. Brett went right back to work helping magicians, musicians, and clowns in many ways. Always problem-solving and creating, Brett tried to find the means to make others succeed in their goals. Whether it was with a retail store, rock band, magician, or clown, Brett stayed busy and made good things happen.

Brett was fascinated at the Patch Adams experience I had the previous September, and seeing his Robyn in her newly found clown role, saw the power of medical clowning first hand. Robyn learned a lot about her new clown character that night in December, and she too was a fan of the Patch Adams movie. She told Brett she wanted a clown lab coat like mine, and he had planned to get one as a surprise for her birthday in July. The months following the holidays were good, and Brett did not show signs of slowing down on any of his projects in spite of his condition, which seemed stable and improving.

Early summer came, and Robyn had arranged a surprise birthday party for Brett. He was looking good, and a great assembly of top magicians in Dallas were there to celebrate his 40th. No one would have ever imagined that Brett had anything wrong with him. Conditions changed very quickly just a few weeks later, and no one expected what was to happen next.

My 50th birthday happened to be just a month later in July, and my wife Darlene had also crafted a well-planned surprise birthday party for me. Under the guise of meeting another couple at my favorite Italian restaurant, I was taken completely off guard when I discovered all my friends and family gathered in a large room. After a short time, I learned that two expected guests were missing. My wife told me Brett and Robyn were supposed to be there. No word for their absence came. I had a sick feeling in my gut, and a quick phone call confirmed my suspicions. Brett was back in the hospital. Robyn said Brett hated to be missing my party and did not want to bring a downer on the day by telling me they were back in the hospital. They assured me he was doing ok and was having a little fever and other symptoms that needed checking. He sounded ok, but the seriousness of his medical issues was just beginning to manifest. I visited him the next day, and then nearly every day afterward. We were back in the fight again at St. Paul Medical Center. This time the gloves were coming off.

I made daily stops at the hospital to offer help as a nurse, clown, or magician and be a support for whatever was needed that day. I worked clinically at a pediatric specialty hospital at Baylor called Our Children's House just a few minutes away and stopping by St. Paul Hospital to see Brett was a great way to wait out Dallas traffic. It was important to me to be available to assist with any medical related conversations, and it is always good to have medical friends around when needed. To help bridge good relationships with the staff and for the pleasure of our enjoyment, I managed to get nearly every member of his medical team to wear clown noses at one time or another whenever lighter moments were timely and desired.

We mostly talked about magic, of course, and I was grateful to have Brett coach me on my favorite routine called Rub a Dub cups and balls right there at his bedside. I learned it from a Bill Malone DVD but had changed the ending of the script to make it more kid friendly. Brett and Bill worked together in years past and were good friends. Brett shared great stories about working with Malone. He is one of my all-time favorite magicians.

Brett appreciated the ease at which I could switch from clown to nurse and back again as the moment required. I tried to offer support to Robyn and his family, at times providing breaks for them to take care of themselves and to assist in their understanding of hospital routines, always seeking to prevent undue anxiety from developing. Being available as a sounding board to help facilitate care planning was appreciated too. Brett was placed high on the transplant list for a liver, and his condition was steadily deteriorating. Every time a new setback emerged, we re-threaded the needle of our medical plan and kept our hope high that a solution would materialize quickly.

Brett maintained his brilliant wit and sense of humor, and we continued our magic talks and planned new goals following the transplant. He was super interested in doing more to help others with his magic. He said that if he made it through this, he wanted to give back to others with his art. His mother Karen later told me that when Brett started out in magic as a kid, he performed his first magic shows in hospitals and nursing homes. She was so supportive of his dreams and very proud of how he wanted to make people happy with magic at a very young age.

Brett's parents Karen and Bob returned again to Dallas, and we all hoped that a donated organ would become available soon. Robyn and her sister Tracy were always there too, praying, nurturing, and believing for healing. No longer the clown, I was just a faithful and supportive friend helping out however I could.

Brett was gravely ill when a liver finally became available. Surgery was scheduled the next morning, and hopes were high that this, the only shot Brett had left, would work. He went to sleep for surgery with courage and hope. Sadly, the damage to other internal organs was worse than expected, and conditions were not favorable for the transplant. It became apparent to all of us Brett's fight was ending. They moved him to the surgical ICU and did everything medically possible to stabilize him in those final hours. Brett left this world with his family at his side. He was surrounded by incredible love when his birthday to Heaven came.

Though Patch could not visit Brett during this time, his phone calls were much appreciated, and his advice to me personally strengthened me to stay positive and be emotionally present for my friend. Clowning was a trick to bring love close, and also to escape from the sadness we were feeling. You know you are loved when your friends are wearing clown noses for you.

Robyn and I found a lot of comfort from those red noses, and we clowned to bring love close to Brett, his nurses, neighboring patients, and anyone we met who needed it. Brett's last gift to Robyn was a clown doctor lab coat like mine that we ordered from Gesundheit Institute. It was going to be a surprise, but it arrived a few days after Brett went to Heaven. I brought it to Robyn's store to present it to her that Saturday morning. The moment I walked in to give it to her, Brett's favorite song began to play on her radio, Matt Redman's 10,000 Reasons. Yes, we cried like babies. Thanks, Sucker Punch.

Robyn, aka Dr. Ra Ra, and I continue to clown together in hospitals, wearing our clown lab coats from Gesundheit. We hope to do as much good as we possibly can through our therapeutic clown and magic work.

The comedy and tragedy masks we associate with theater signify the enduring struggle between light and dark, joy and sorrow, life and death. We cannot let sadness dominate our stage for very long. The show must go on.

Brett Wolf would have insisted upon it.

Magic Nurse — Bedside Artist

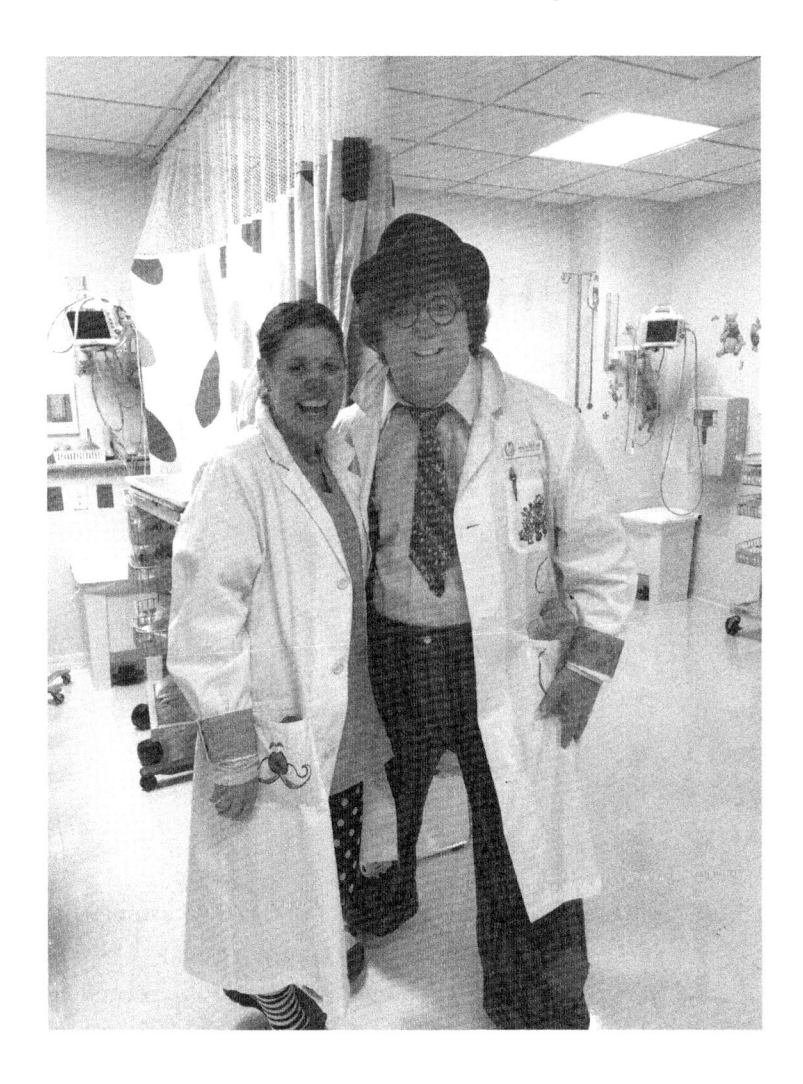

CHAPTER 9
MAGIC AS THERAPY

"I do believe in an everyday sort of magic—the inexplicable connectedness we sometimes experience with places, people, works of art and the like; the eerie appropriateness of moments of synchronicity; the whispered voice, the hidden presence, when we think we are alone."

—*Charles de Lint*

MAGICIANS ARE KEENLY FAMILIAR WITH the astonishment effect magic has on spectators, and that sense of wonder has as much benefit as humor does in a healing experience. Just as medical clowns, humor, and music therapies have found their way into clinical environments, the idea of performance magic as a therapeutic activity has brought professional magic entertainers into the medical environment to partner with therapists in helping patients with physical and occupational therapy goals.

The 1006-page magic book copyrighted in 1938, *Greater Magic* by John Northern Hilliard [9] is considered a classic and essential to a magician's personal library. This book is about the size of a cinder block and contains over 1150 illustrations by Harlan Tarbell, who authored an eight-volume complete course in performance magic titled *Tarbell Course in Magic*. [10] These two works alone contain more than any single magician could use in a lifetime, yet these are only considered a good start in the library of a serious student of magic. With a history that dates back to biblical times, the origins of magic had a high value in ancient societies and numerous cultures throughout human history. Moses faced off with the Pharaoh's magicians who, with their clever illusions, did not have a prayer against the divine power of the Almighty.

Tarbell reveals in volume one of his magic course that medicine in its earliest form was rooted in magic, in the practice of shamans, priests, and magicians.

"The most primitive method of treating disease was the use of spells and incantations by the magician," Harlan writes. "Then came the use of stones, sticks, and strings to draw out diseases."

He goes on to describe how elixirs, ointments, and the use of herbs followed, which branched off into the beginnings of pharmacology. From these early beginnings, medicine evolved out of the realms of superstition and magical potions to a practice based in sciences as did every other advancement of knowledge. Apparently, the use of the magician in the early civilizations provided a placebo effect in making the patient believe something was going to happen. If it did not turn out well, then recovery was just not in the stars nor favored by the gods. Chance and fate left the magician blameless, unlike our modern-day doctors who risk lawsuits daily.

Today, we understand that magic has always been a clever ruse. Performances appear to alter reality, accomplished by the hidden talents of the magician. This performance art has entertainment value so long as a suspension of disbelief is present. Magicians have always been actors with the added benefit of a craft that uses specially engineered devices, props, and tools to create an illusion that appears as an impossible reality. The sudden impossibility produces a moment of astonishment, which is a very powerful response to create in another person. Fooling entire populations resulted as many Emperors, Kings, and Pharaohs had their court of magicians working to assist wherever magical revelation or divine illusion was helpful to rule.

Stepping into the modern world, we enjoy magic entertainment as the performing art that it is. What often begins as a childhood hobby can continue throughout a lifetime for a budding young magician. As a spectator, we all will stop and watch a magician whenever they catch our attention with an incredible effect. We cannot help but have some emotional response to it. Our curiosity is too great to ignore what the eyes are seeing. When magic finds its way into hospitals and shares visual impossibilities with patients, a moment of wonder and astonishment occurs. I have personally seen the beauty of its gifts in many magical encounters.

As a close-up magician, I bring a new game into the care relationship. At the right moments and under the right circumstances, a magic trick can also be used to empower patients when we teach the method to those who desire to participate. Magic is enjoyed both as a spectator and a student, depending on the desires and imaginations of the patients. Whether used for entertainment or therapy, magic has an important place in the art of medicine, and I'd like to share with you two very special programs that I champion in my work that bring magic therapy to the bedside and teach this beautiful art.

David Copperfield and Kevin Spencer are pioneers in the development of using performance magic in therapeutic ways. David's book *Project Magic Handbook* [11] is considered the first of its kind in therapeutic magic, and Kevin's Healing of Magic [12] and Hocus Focus [13] curriculum are bringing this art into therapy programs around the world.

Copperfield wrote, "As a person with a disability learns the mechanics of a magical illusion, they are motivated to increase physical dexterity, functional skills, and communication. ... Self-esteem and motivation are essential to the achievement of rehabilitation goals." [14]

Early in my magic nursing journey, I became friends with Kevin Spencer and studied his Healing of Magic program, which he was actively teaching in seminars and workshops around the world. I added his methods to my practice, adapted and facilitated this program as a volunteer magician to assist physical and occupational therapists, recreational therapists, and child life specialists. Kevin is a true champion of integrating magic as a therapeutic modality and continues to develop this work into new areas. The latest, and I believe his greatest work yet, is his Hocus Focus program. The successes he has witnessed, especially with autistic kids, has been phenomenal.

Kevin travels extensively, teaching and conducting workshops and seminars with medical and educational professionals all over the globe. He and his beautiful wife Cindy have dedicated their lives to helping others with magic therapy methods. He has taken magic therapy further than anyone could have imagined. I asked Kevin what got him started in magic and how that evolved into his therapeutic magic mission and if he would mind sharing his vision with us for this book. He was glad to help.

Here is his story:

> My name is Kevin Spencer, and I am a performing artist. When I was five years old, I saw a magician perform on television and remember vividly telling my mom, "When I grow up, I'm going to be a magician!" My parents bought me a magic kit at age eight, and I worked hard on each of those tricks, performing them for friends and family.
>
> In the seventh grade, my focus changed from magic to music, and for the next several years, I worked on becoming a concert pianist. That is until Doug Henning arrived on the scene. Henning revived my fascination with magic. My love of magic and music continued through college.
>
> During one of my breaks from college, I went home to visit my parents in Indiana and was fortunate to see Doug Henning perform live at the Holiday Star Theatre

in Merrillville. In hopes of getting a chance to meet Doug in person, I wrote a note and passed it to an usher before the show. He assured me he would get it to him, then returned later to tell me that it might be possible to meet Mr. Henning at the stage door following the show.

I was ecstatic!

Arriving at the backstage door, I found hundreds of people also waiting to see Doug Henning. I learned that several others also sent notes asking for a chance to meet, so I thought I would not get an opportunity after all and decided to start the long drive home. As I was working my way out of the crowd, Henning's road manager came out and asked, "Is Kevin Spencer in the crowd?" I identified myself and was told, "Mr. Henning would like to see you in his dressing room." I was stunned. I spent over an hour talking with him about touring with a large production and life on the road. He was warm and personable, just as he was on stage. It was an extraordinary experience and one I will never forget!

Fast forward to several years later as Cindy and I began to develop our illusion production. Having only been married a few years, our lives were changed dramatically. As a result of a near-fatal car accident, I suffered a closed head injury and lower spinal cord injury. I spent the next several months in physical and occupational therapy, aware that I might never perform again. During that time, I realized how challenging it is for a patient to stay motivated during long-term rehabilitation. Once I regained function, Cindy and I collaborated with therapists to develop a program that would use simple magic tricks to help regain lost physical skills while increasing motivational levels and self-esteem. This is the foundation of the Healing of Magic.

Over the years, I've learned so much about people with different abilities. My own process of recovery was challenging. It gave me a greater appreciation for what people with disabilities deal with every day of their lives. We think they are different than the rest of us. They're not. They have hopes and dreams just like you and me, but their futures are often molded by the attitudes and perceptions we have about them. As a society, it's time for us to start appreciating what they can do and stop focusing on what we believe they can't do.

Today, the concepts of magic therapy are being used in more than 2000 hospitals, rehabilitation facilities, and schools in over 30 countries. I earned the Approved Provider status of the American Occupational Therapy Association and certification in Autism Studies. My work is focused on researching arts-integrated interventions for clients and providing relevant, useful, and engaging continuing education for therapists and educators.

— Kevin Spencer

Visit http://www.magictherapy.com/ for more information and program details.

Kevin and I have had many conversations about our practice of magic in clinical settings. My favorite use of his program was in my volunteer work with the Spina Bifida Association of North Texas. For several years, I provided medical first aid at Camp John Marc in Meridian, TX, which is an extraordinary place that hosts several weeklong and weekend camps for children with a variety of medical conditions. As a camp nurse, I had the joy of using this venue to empower my kids with learning sleight of hand magic tricks both from Kevin's curriculum and my personal favorite effects.

Year after year, I continue to add new magic, and now include circus skills like scarf juggling, plate spinning, ribbon dancing, and feather balancing to my therapeutic play. I continue to explore new arts like cartooning, origami, and improvisation games, which also have therapeutic value.

I was so lucky to find a great magician like Kevin to guide me. The motivational effects and enhancement of self-esteem through Healing of Magic methods are clearly evident and long lasting for the kids. Whenever a child is motivated and challenged to achieve attainable goals and gain new skills, real magic happens!

CHAPTER 10

DREAM DOCTOR PROJECT - MEDICAL CLOWNS IN ACTION

"The role of the Clown and the Physician are the same- it's to elevate the possible and to relieve suffering."

— *Patch Adams*

I CONSIDER MYSELF A CLINICAL PERFORMING Artist because I have integrated several types of performance art into my clinical practice. Music, magic, and therapeutic clown arts are all now part of the journey, and the skills from each have a place in hospital work. As a working nurse, I watch for the most valuable opportunity to use whatever talent is best suited for each situation. I studied the best medical clowning programs in the world and recently talked with Michael Christensen, who is the founder of the Big Apple Circus Clown Care program started in 1986 here in America. [15]

Big Apple medical clowns make nearly 225,000 visits to young patients in sixteen leading pediatric facilities each year across the United States. Considered the Godfather of medical clowning, Michael Christensen travels all over the world providing lectures and workshops in the unique art of medical clowning. As we talked about the differences in various programs during a recent phone call, he was very passionate about the growth of medical clowning as a profession throughout the world. He spoke very highly of the Dream Doctor Project in Israel specifically, where he has lectured often. [16] He shared his thoughts on the unique qualities that make the program in Israel so successful. I went to Israel in 2014 to shadow several clowns, train with the Dream Doctors, and experience for myself their specialized program.

The Dream Doctor Project began in 2002 in Hadassah Hebrew University Hospital in Jerusalem and has grown to partner with 29 hospitals throughout Israel, with more than 111 official paid professional medical clown positions. Dream Doctors visit approximately 200,000 adults and children each year. The Dream Doctor Project has led the way in research in this field. In the area of medical clown research, they write:

"In 2011, the Dream Doctors Project First International Conference on Medicine and Medical Clowning was held in Jerusalem. We hosted 250 guests from 22 countries, including medical clowns, representatives of medical clowning associations from around the world, and physicians and nurses. Several medical studies on the issue of medical clowning were presented, making it clear that there was a need for additional scientific studies to form an evidence-based foundation for medical clowns' contribution to patient wellbeing and health. Consequently, the conference resolved to establish a Scientific Research Fund to provide grants each year for research on medical clowning. Prof. Arthur Eidelman is chairman of the Scientific Committee, which so far has supported twenty-two articles on various topics in the field of medical clowning." [17]

Tsour Shriqui, Director of the Dream Doctor Project, shared with me an essential quality that makes their program so effective:

"The work of the Dream Doctor clowns, as we see it, is beyond humor," he said. "The clown is not a visitor in the hospital who comes to entertain the children. He is part of the medical team."

The formula for the success of this program is in the sound principles it has developed:

The Vision:

"We are working to promote medical clowning as an officially recognized paraprofessional medical profession recognized through proper academic training so that each child in the hospital will have the advantage of benefiting from the encounter with a Dream Doctor."

The Project Goals:

1. Motivate the child patient to address the illness and empower the child in the coping process.
2. Alleviate the hospitalization experience for the patient's family.
3. Become fully integrated into the care processes as part of the multisystemic care staff to move the treatment forward.
4. Add to the scientific foundation and advance a research-oriented scientific community on the issue of medical clowning.
5. Develop an academic curriculum for medical clown training.
6. Advance and develop medical clowning to achieve its official recognition as an official, salaried paramedical profession [18]

Early September 2014, I made my trip to Israel just a few days after a lasting ceasefire was brokered with the Palestinians. I was glad the rocket attacks had stopped and would not be a problem during the two weeks I would tour the country. I partnered with medical clowns in several hospitals in Jerusalem, Afula, and Tel Aviv, as a guest medical clown of the Dream Doctor Project.

During the hostilities, many of the hospital clowns pulled double duty by also visiting bomb shelters to alleviate the stress of children and families confined there during the numerous rocket attacks. Though I came to study their methods of hospital clowning and learn from the best clown therapists in the country, I was impressed by the flexibility these Dream Doctor clowns had for adapting to the needs of children in whatever stressful situation they were experiencing. The clowns also ministered to children outside the hospital, under hostile and dangerous circumstances.

This dedication is a hallmark of the level of commitment and professionalism the Dream Doctor Project clowns have. In May 2015, a team of Dream Doctor clowns went to Nepal following the earthquake there. Israel's IDF (Israeli Defense Force) Medical unit was deployed there to provide medical and surgical care. Joining them in the effort was a team of five medical clowns from the Dream Doctor Project. The clowns integrated with the field hospital staff to relieve stress and anxiety and provide healing and playful joy to the children and adults being treated for their injuries. This inclusion of medical clowns in a disaster zone is truly the highest level of performing art I can imagine.

I was very fortunate to have worked with one of those clowns, Smadar Harpak, at her home hospital Ichilov, in Tel Aviv. She is one of a kind. The response to this tragic event gave us a glimpse at the possibilities for medical clowns. The example set by the Dream Doctor Project to respond in other parts of the world opened a door for this new profession to break new ground, responding as part of disaster relief wherever help is needed.

In the two weeks of my visit with the Dream Doctor Project, I worked in several hospitals as a medical clown with some of the very best therapy clowns in the world. In Jerusalem, I spent a day with Sigalit, working with the physical therapists, and learned how to create clown games to encourage specific physical therapy goals for patients to achieve. A quick report from the physical therapist to inform me of what activity the patient was to perform, then the therapeutic clown brain kicks in to create a fun way to make that happen. Encouraging a little Russian girl bound in full body braces to walk across the room with a walker several times might be considered dreadful if it were not turned into a fun game to play with a clown. Her mother delighted as she watched us work together. This level of therapy and art was exactly the magic I hoped to find on this journey.

I worked with Sigalit helping several patients as they came into the therapy room each hour that day. Working directly with the patients at the direction of the physical therapist made the effectiveness of the therapy easy to accomplish, all the while we elevated the spirits of the child to enjoy interactive play therapy. This result clearly was the dream these clown doctors had in mind when they created the Dream Doctor Project: Empowering the child through therapeutic play to meet therapeutic goals.

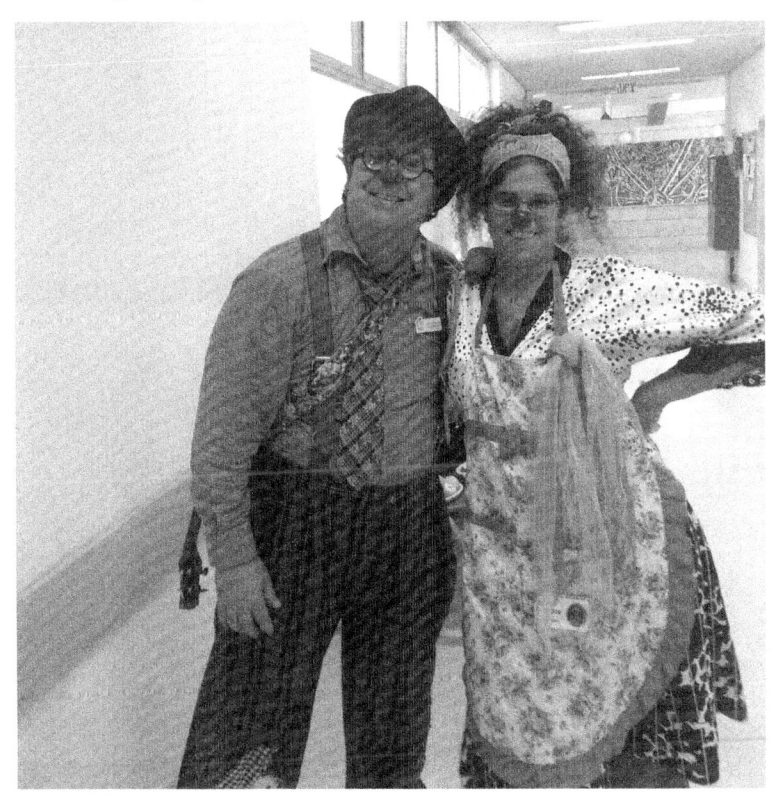

After my time in Jerusalem, I traveled to Haifa to stay for my next visit to another hospital in Afula the following morning. I met a clown named Miki at HaEmek Hospital. Miki was a professional dancer and actor turned medical clown, and we had a fantastic time together. We performed in several areas of the hospital, but the most rewarding times were the adults in the dialysis unit.

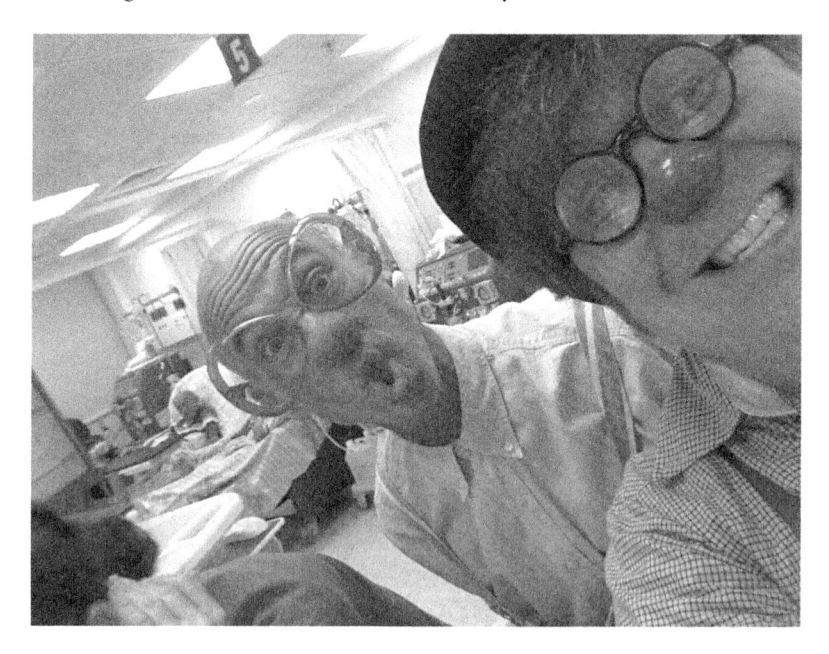

We experienced 'theater in the round'—a circular stage—in this larger room with patients all the way around the perimeter receiving dialysis for several hours. This group was quite the captive audience of adults who also appreciated the therapeutic entertainment clowns bring. Often these patients visit this unit a few days a week for about 4 hours each visit. The hospital performer has to be quite skilled with improvisation and offer new material to keep each encounter fresh. Miki was a master of connection as he shared quality time with each of these patients.

The diversity of cultures all gathered together in this unit was very interesting. Miki pointed out that these patients represented seven different cultures and languages, putting their differences aside to receive much-needed medical care they each required. They would also share the experience of humor, singing, and comedy to heal their spirits. I found that by making napkin roses and singing Elvis songs on the ukulele, I too connected beyond culture differences and found adult clowning to be just as appreciated and relevant in any language. I was so thankful to Miki for sharing so much of his remarkable work with me and letting me experience adult medical clowning with his regular patients. I could see he cared deeply for them.

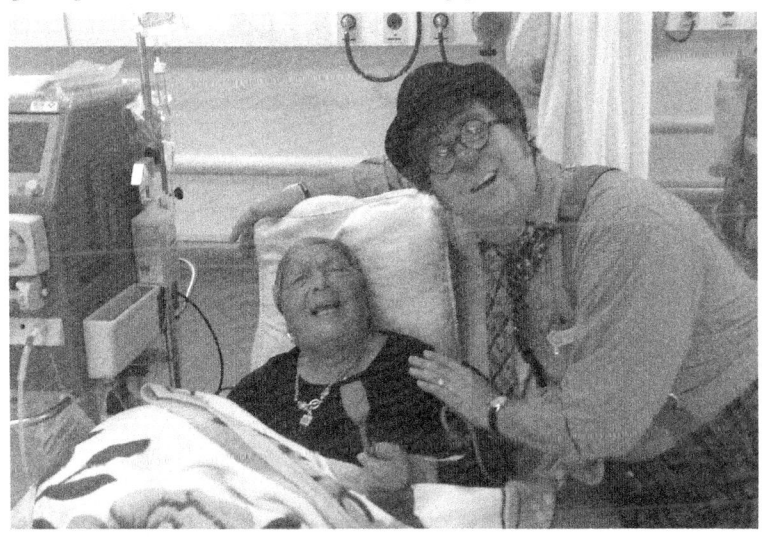

Once in Tel Aviv, I spent the next several days visiting two major hospitals, Mier Medical Center and Ichilov Medical Center. I was so thrilled to meet all the Dream Doctor clowns at their annual celebration of Rosh Hashanah at a special dinner held for them. I had the privilege of meeting the founders of the Dream Doctor project and visited with many clowns who worked throughout Israel. I was privileged to share some therapeutic magic effects I used with many of the clowns and made lasting friendships I cherish today. Karin was my guide throughout my time in Israel and had arranged many experiences that have influenced my work so profoundly. Karin invited me to attend the opening night of a remarkable play about medical clowning from the perspective of the clown's inner thoughts. It was an original dramatic play that brought me to tears it was so powerful. Karin translated the Hebrew dialogue in whispers for me, and the entire experience at the Arab-Hebrew Theatre in Jaffa that night will stay with me always.

In Tel Aviv the next day, I worked with an amazing clown at Ichilov, Smadar Harpak, aka "Shamash" which means "Sunshine" in Hebrew. Having been one of the clowns who visited bomb shelters, her gifts were valued wherever she went. Later in 2015, her work in Nepal would again be a testament to her dedication to using her arts to heal.

Magic Nurse — Bedside Artist

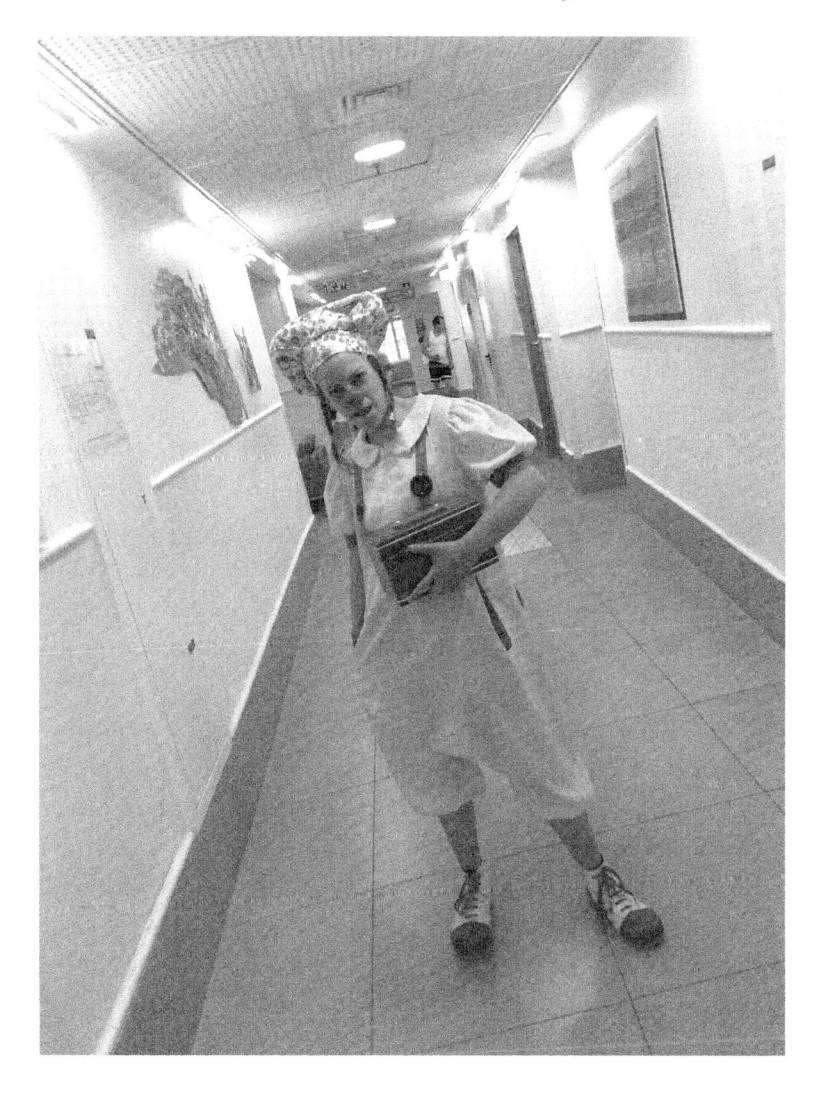

When we met that morning, I immediately felt her incredible energy. We visited several units and had several patient experiences together. She had a keen sense of her patient's mood, and engaged them with care, connecting with such comedic grace. It was heartwarming seeing her work. We learned as much as we could from each other during our day. Afterward, we had lunch at her favorite local cafe, where I listened with amazement at her stories of clowning adventures. Smadar is also an accomplished actress and performer outside her hospital work. She truly is a medical clown superhero in my book!

I spent my last hospital day with Penny Hanuka at Meir Medical Center. Penny wrote a great deal of the clowning procedures and approaches taught to Dream Doctor clowns. She is well traveled and academically trained for this work. She is also deeply involved in Dream Doctors research studies to help establish medical clowning as a para-medicine. Anyone can visit their website to learn about medical clowning, and there are numerous research studies and articles written on key aspects of medical clown work.

Performing as a clown partner with Penny on that last hospital day was the capstone of my education on this mission. She had a great deal of medical knowledge blended into her thoughtful clown technique; I knew I was working with possibly the best medical clown instructor in the world. From a clinical perspective, she could have easily been a medical professional herself. With her use of clowning technique, in such a precise manner, I felt a clinical connection to her clown style that defined this important truth:

Medical clowning, at its highest form of expression, is just as necessary as nurses and doctors in the healthcare environment.

Through my time with Penny, I was able to see what kind of clown I was aspiring to become. I came from a medical profession into the world of medical clowning and was fusing my inherent artistic abilities with my nursing skills. I recognized these same qualities in Penny, as she had mastered the therapeutic value of this higher level of medical clowning and already was a champion of this most unusual work. I cannot thank Penny, Dvorit, and the other wonderful clowns at Meir enough for sharing so much of their talents and skills in our time together. I would love to have stayed longer!

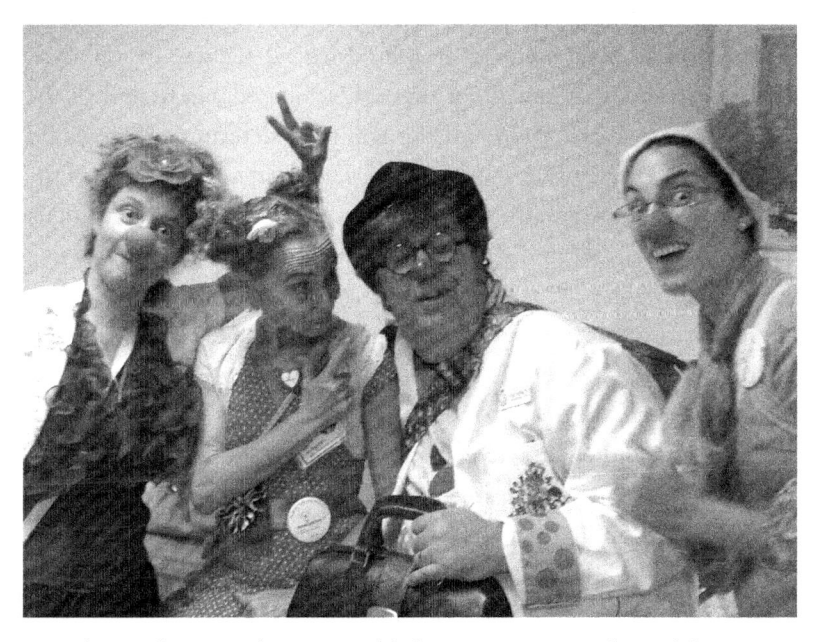

I learned as much as I could during my time there. There is no formal way to get the training needed to integrate all that is necessary to be an expert medical clown as the profession is still in its infancy. Collaboration and mentoring seem to be the best way to gain the skills for this specialized craft. Unlike magic, there are no books available that take medical clowning education to its highest potential. Magic has thousands of books written over hundreds of years available. Medical clowning has only just begun with relatively few masters of the craft. Seeking out these pioneers and learning from them is vital to growing this field of medical clown work.

I reached out to some of my Dream Doctor friends one year after my visit to get some additional insight to share in this book, and I continue to find new discoveries of the value of this work. Penny responded and shared some new developments in the area of sedation for procedures and diagnostics. This use of clown as a substitute for sedation is an area of particular interest to me since I worked as a pediatric sedation nurse for several years.

Penny was lecturing for doctors and nurses in a professional sedation course being offered at Meir Medical Center in Tel Aviv. She told me about the idea that through a focused assessment of the emotional state of the child and the family to determine if the child could become cooperative with the encouragement and guidance of the medical clown to negate the need for sedation drugs. By establishing a connection of trust with the clown and reducing the stress and fear of a procedure through playful education, many children find the ability and willingness to cooperate and subsequently achieve an accomplishment that reinforces empowerment and self-esteem. The important thing is to create a connection at the beginning with actions that reduce stress and fear and elicit active cooperation. Strengthening the child's therapeutic space before, during, and following the procedure will give the child the capability to cope, and thereby eliminate fear and anxiety, replacing it with fun and empowerment. Penny continues to provide training and research and is a real champion of this profession.

As a sedation nurse, I used similar approaches whenever assessing a child that had the potential to cooperate if given the opportunity to be encouraged before proceeding with sedation. A CT scan only takes a few minutes if the child could be still. If sedation were needed, they would be with me for an hour or two more until discharge, and feel hung-over for the rest of the day. Whenever I could reduce the time for my patients, my department benefited from the time returned to our schedule to serve more patients waiting for scans. The patient's experience is much more pleasant when no drugs are needed.

It begins by engaging and having a dialogue with the child to let them express themselves about their fears, and to create a trusting relationship where the child feels able to learn and sample the experience in a friendly way. Often we would make it a game, and with games, there was now fun attached. Whatever it took to make it fun is what I did. Staying with the child and parent, we played together and shared in the small victory when the child accomplished the procedure or study on their own, without medication.

Penny says the medical staff is very receptive to the work of the medical clowns at Meir and continue to contribute to the successful integration of this artistic and creative approach to caring for the child. Penny told me she hopes we in America would have this level of cooperation, too. Attracting serious attention to this medical clown profession would begin to see positive results for the lives of hospitalized children everywhere.

Gabriel Bartra is another great medical clown friend from Israel. He has been a medical clown for eleven years at the time of this writing. His clown name is Dr. Pepe. Coming from a career in radio production, he wanted to learn more about acting and trained in clown and physical arts. Through a colleague, he heard of the Dream Doctor Project and became a medical clown.

When asked about the most rewarding aspect of this work, Gabriel said, "Helping to change the perception of clowning as a way to alleviate stress and anxiety. Helping others to release whatever tensions they have is what medical clowns are best at.

"To the nurses and doctors I would like to say, feel free to express yourself! Let us help support your work. As an artist, we can help provide the emotional care in cooperation with your healing effort. Our work is very complimentary to each other in the hospital. A doctor or nurse can play along with us too!

"In life, there is a role for everyone and the ones who compliment you are the ones who are there to help you reach your goals and dreams."

Today there are medical clown programs in several countries, and the profession is expanding and growing in many places throughout the world, we could do better at home in America though. The Associated Press recently reported that it became law in Argentina that children's hospitals must provide specially trained clowns as part of their healthcare facilities. In the USA, there are only a handful of paid therapeutic clown programs at children's hospitals, and virtually nothing in community hospitals that serve both adults and children. We have no shortage of volunteer clowns willing to visit and entertain, but the higher skills needed for therapeutic work is hard to acquire. We have a long way to go and much we can learn from our friends in Israel. I would like to do something about this, sooner rather than later!

I have studied many of the Dream Doctor Project's posted articles and watched several of their lectures from experts in this field from around the world. If I could have only one dream come true, it would be to see Dream Doctors come to America to inspire creativity and new ideas to help us redesign our healthcare delivery system. I dream for hospitals everywhere to be more loving, creative, nurturing, and kind to our people, young and old.

CHAPTER 11

FLOWER POWER: THE MAGIC OF A ROSE

"I will soothe you and heal you. I will bring you roses. I too have been covered with thorns."

—*Rumi*

Though I had not directly intended to invoke the images of Berkeley in the 1960s with this chapter title, I could not help but appreciate the time in our history where the words "flower power" represented the love revolution in American culture. As groovy and exciting as the peace movement might be to talk about, it is not the direction I was going. (I was only six years old when Woodstock happened.) Instead, I am going to share the tender moments I have personally discovered through the use of a particular flower made from a simple paper napkin. You can transform any simple square napkin into a token of loving action.

This chapter is about paper roses made with love, and the healing powers we have discovered by making them and giving them away. There is a particular product I use to make flowers for my patients, which creates a unique moment in the hospital that is always appreciated by patients and their families. You can provide both a simple act of kindness and a heartwarming bedside performance when you make a paper rose for a patient. A small handmade memento to lift the spirits. Giving paper roses to patients has been the most powerful moments of connection I have experienced in my work as a clinical artist. You can easily do this too. These roses have a unique quality and might be the best tool I have found for creating a healing performance that will last long after we leave the patient's bedside.

I first learned of napkin roses at a clown convention, demonstrated to me by an excellent professional clown, J T "Bubba" Sikes. He told me how valuable the roses have been in his work as a hospital clown and it only took five minutes to instruct me on the finer points of making them. This uniquely designed napkin square with perfectly colored printing to make a colored rose blossom with green stems was cool, and I made a beautiful red rose on my first attempt.

This napkin rose became one of my favorite clinical props for the hospital in a very short time. I purchased a large quantity in several colors of these specially designed napkins and began using them regularly. I soon discovered several powerful applications these props offered in hospital clown and magic visits. Not only a great prop for performance pieces, but they also provided therapeutic opportunity to teach and empower patients to share in the creative exercise of making their own flowers. Frequently I would bring a dozen roses (actually, a short stack of colored napkins) and the patient and I would make a few together at first so they could learn the skill and continue making them after I left. Paper flowers were especially nice for patients who were unable to have fresh flowers in their rooms due to weakened immunities and the risk of infection live plants present. Paper roses became a great substitute and the act of creating them at the bedside made for many wonderful patient experiences.

There is not a single encounter in my experience where the napkin rose did not deliver a great result. I imagine it's because flowers have been a means to express love for centuries. It is practically an expectation that when a friend or loved one becomes hospitalized, we are quick to send flowers to show that our thoughts, prayers, and love are with them. It is certainly within the scope of any caregiver's practice to join in with families and friends to show support and encouragement too. Flowers make patients feel better.

Teaching this fast-learned form of origami to patients is also offered as a shared experience, it opens doors to other priceless empowering moments. I have been witness to wonderfully loving exchanges when a husband lying in a hospital bed had an opportunity to give a flower he made to his beloved wife, who was tirelessly attending him at his bedside. The power to give is often more necessary than to receive. I have taught patients how to make roses to give to their favorite nurses, doctors, or anyone else they wished. Aside from the nurse call button and the TV remote, making roses is a powerful tool for patients. The flower is a vehicle and a means to allow patients to connect with others on a friendly level. I know for a fact that when patients make paper roses for their nurses, they are treasured by their caregivers.

The patient-caregiver relationship improves when these types of connections happen in a healing environment. The positive energy flows in two directions and makes being a caregiver a real privilege. Naturally, all the expected professionalism should be maintained in every clinical practice, though I suspect an over-strict application of professional distance might contribute to what is wrong with the growing dissatisfaction we have in healthcare. It is possible and highly desired to be genuinely more caring in our actions while being professional in our practice. There is a lot we can do at the bedside to make the patient experience more human.

Looking back at the many patient encounters I had making roses, I realized I had to share the impact this simple paper napkin made. My personal experiences were so memorable they deserved more than a side mention. I felt a chapter dedicated to "The Rose" would encourage clinicians to adopt this performance tool for themselves to share in their clinical practices. If every nurse learned this one simple craft and used it in their work, they will have gained a new "Superpower" to create happy moments for themselves and their patients.

When I thought about where to start in this chapter, I contacted the creator of this product, Michael Mode, magician, corporate trainer, and owner of Big Lightbulb Inc., to learn how he came up with this great idea. We became fast friends as we shared many similar stories of the magic these roses have created around the world. He impressed me so, I knew I had to ask him to tell his story too. Michael's journey into magic is fascinating, and the creation of this simple product has taken on a life of its own. His story moved me. Michael has been quite humbled also, and surprised by the many stories shared with him about the impact this product has made. Flower Power is about the magic of love!

Here is the backstory Michael shared for this chapter:

> When I debuted Napkin Roses as a product back in 2004, I never imagined that years later I would be asked to write about them for a book. The thought never even crossed my mind that these simple napkin origami roses would be used all over the world in hospitals and countless other places to help make memories and bring smiles to the faces of those in need. The success of napkin roses has exceeded my wildest expectations and the experiences they have provided me over the past dozen years have been very rewarding and humbling.
>
> When I was a young child, my mother took me out for dinner at a restaurant in our hometown of Detroit. While we were eating, a waiter twisted a rose out of a white cocktail napkin. I was fascinated by this simple creation, but didn't learn how to make one of my own until quite a few years later when I became interested in magic.
>
> I started performing magic professionally when I was thirteen. I worked at quite a few restaurants during high school and college and would make roses out of napkins from time to time to hand out as a special souvenir for

guests on Valentine's Day or other special events like a birthday or anniversary. The reaction to the roses was always fantastic, often generating better reactions than the magic I performed, so I continued to make them and hand them out.

I knew other magicians were making the paper roses and had heard they were also popular with waiters and bartenders, especially on cruise ships. One day, I had the thought of a rose made out of a napkin that was two-toned so that the flower would be red and the stem would be green. I wrote the thought down in a notebook but didn't pursue the idea any further at the time.

Around 2003, I started thinking about a red and green napkin rose again and decided to search for napkin companies online. After contacting nearly 100 companies and learning quite a bit about how napkins are made and printed, I gave up on the idea. It turned out there were quite a few printing issues to overcome, and none of the manufacturers were as interested in the idea as I was. Most companies wouldn't even return my calls or emails.

A year later, I decided to revisit the idea and contacted more manufacturers. My diligence paid off when I found one napkin manufacturer who agreed to pursue the project with me. The only catch was that I had to order 65,000 red/green napkins! Also, since the printing plates had to be created, I was placing the order without seeing a sample of the product to make sure it would work as I imagined. After some consideration, I bit the bullet, paid the money, and ordered 65,000 custom printed napkins…sight unseen!

I'll never forget the feeling I had that day the semi-truck backed up to my condo with the long-awaited delivery. My friend Keith came over to help me unload the pallets full of napkins, and I kept thinking to myself, *This is either going to be really great or I'm going to have red and green Christmas napkins for the rest of my life!*

It turns out the napkins were great and worked just as I had imagined for twisting a red and green rose. I introduced the napkins for the first time in August of 2004 at a magic convention, the Abbott's Magic Get-Together in Colon, Michigan. They were a huge hit with magicians, and I sold out of the initial batch shortly after. A couple of orders later, I decided to print some pink/green and yellow/green napkins, and then a year later, added white/green and purple/green.

Fast forward a dozen years and the stories about napkin roses continue to amaze me. One time, a girl told me her father made napkin roses for all of the women at his office. Later that evening, he surprised his wife with two dozen napkin roses when she came home from work. Sadly, the man passed away two weeks later. It turns out the napkin roses were the last flowers he ever gave his wife! At his funeral, the women from his office mentioned that they would always keep those flowers as a fond memory of him. Wow!

Even the Red Cross uses napkin roses in times of tragedy to help people take their minds off the situation at hand. Napkin roses were handed out to the first responders, teachers, and parents after the Sandy Hook school shooting a few years ago. All of this is just mind-boggling to me as I never imagined them being used in these ways.

More often, napkin roses are handed out during happy times. Teachers make them with their students, churches use them to highlight lessons, and many people have used them during marriage proposals. People keep these napkin roses forever.

I've made a lot of friends as a direct result of these napkins. Whenever people tell me about the results they get from using them, I am always delighted and humbled. When Rob contacted me to let me know about writing this book, we had never met or talked before. An hour later, we were instant friends as he shared the amazing stories of the good work he does in hospitals and the role that napkin roses along with magic and humor play in his daily visits with patients.

My favorite saying is, "You never know when you're making a memory."

The more I've thought about those words over the years, the more I realize how true they really are. *You never know when you're making a memory.*

When I was very young, that waiter who made the rose out of the white napkin for my mother made a memory with me. That inspired me to make roses of my own, which led me to the idea of manufacturing multi-colored napkins to make more realistic napkin roses.

My mother taught me many wonderful lessons over the years and remains my biggest influence. Unfortunately, she never got to see my version of the napkin rose because she passed away almost ten years before I had them manufactured. My most successful product to date is based on a rose. Ironically, my mother's name was also Rose.

I hope the napkin roses help you create many memories of your own.

— Michael Mode [19]

Thanks to the vision of my friend Michael, I made the napkin rose discovery in my nursing practice. You do not have to be a magician or a clown to take this simple skill and run with it to your heart's delight. The smallest gesture can have the biggest impact. We have all experienced moments like that in our lives. If you haven't, try making a rose for a patient and you will feel the power too.

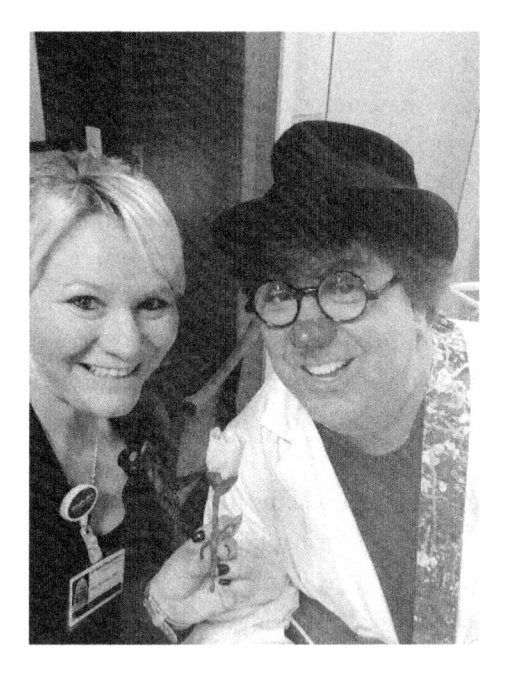

CHAPTER 12

NOT JUST A NURSE

"You're going to be there when a lot of people are born, and when a lot of people die. In most every culture, such moments are regarded as sacred and private, made special by a divine presence. No one on Earth would be welcomed, but you're personally invited. What an honor that is."

– Thom Dick

I HAVE SHARED MY CLINICAL ARTISTIC journey and the unexpected twists and turns I discovered along the way. The details of my story are unique to me, but the intent, compassion, and drive are a common trait among many nurses. I learned how to connect with my patients using close-up magic and improvisational humor, which have proven to be useful tools in my approach to nursing care. Each nurse must find their own unique super power.

Nurses relieve the suffering of others. We follow the rules and standards of our practice while dutifully supporting doctors in theirs. We are educators, advocates, and therapists. We tend to physical, emotional, spiritual, and psychological needs. We are comforters, prayer warriors, and friends. We use every one of our God-given talents in our profession, and our natural place is at the bedside, inches away from our patients.

All nurses know and use traditional comfort measures, and many also draw on their own personal talents and gifts to create meaningful care relationships. Simply taking the time to sit, listen, and talk *with* your patients as opposed to talking *at them* is a valuable skill for beginning a care partnership. Nurses who have their heart committed to the call of this profession easily find the "extra stuff" in themselves. Your personal bedside manner is an expression of who you are.

Be physically and intellectually present for those persons entrusted to your care. Focus and make use of every one of your human senses in every patient encounter. Listen to the irregular beats of damaged hearts. Hear the wheezing and crackles in straining lungs, the grumbling in bellies, and anxiety in whispering voices. See the emotions expressed in tear-filled eyes, trembling, pain, and restlessness in weak and failing bodies. With Your hands, feel the heat from fevers, the coldness of deprived circulation when massaging sore muscles, applying balms, lotions, ointments, and bandages to fragile skin. Therapeutic touch is a means to comfort our patients and assure them they are not alone.

When we consider the entire healthcare system from a distant and objective view, we lose sight of what I believe is the most important element of it: the experience of the person looking outward from their hospital bed. Not until you physically find yourself in a hospital bed, will you notice that your field of view narrows so that you think less about the bigger issues. What becomes most important is the relationships you have with others, especially your nurse.

The very first time I considered becoming a nurse was at a time when a very compassionate and plain speaking hospice nurse came into my father's home to help him live out his last few days in his battle with pancreatic cancer. Our family was close at hand, and a hospital bed was set up in the living room so Dad could be in his own home with familiar surroundings. She was a welcomed guest, and our gratitude for her compassionate care was immeasurable. She taught us about what was happening and guided our understanding of everything. She took care of the medical needs of a dying man while preserving his and our humanity. We were able to share that time as a family, surrounding ourselves with love, with a nurse at our side as my father, fully aware and cognitive to his last breath, mouthed the words "I love you" to my mother before he closed his eyes for the last time. I never considered that our nurse had seen this transition from life countless times because this was our first, and she was everything we needed during a time when we were helpless and afraid. She was not just a nurse; she was *our* nurse.

I witnessed an awakening of sorts in the nursing profession as Miss Colorado, Kelley Johnson, RN, walked out on the Miss America Pageant stage in her hospital scrubs to share her most precious talents with America in 2015. [20] Kelley verbalized a heartwarming experience that was her defining example of the "extra stuff" nurses use in their professional practice. The power to connect to another human being by whatever means necessary to lift them up from their distress. In her experience, Kelley saw the actual nature of care as her patient likewise treated her. Care went both ways in this exchange. Her talent was the ability to communicate as she held her patient's hand and looked into his eyes, talking to him like he was a person and not a diagnosis. This connection is the real magic of nursing.

Caring is bidirectional: it goes in two directions when both caregiver and patient engage with each other. Joe was just as willing to offer care to the nurse as she was present and able to provide it. Both people had something to offer each other.

Kelley was moved by her patient encounter and told her story to America on national television. She could have sung a song, twirled a baton, or rocked out some dance moves for the pageant. Instead, she gave nursing the limelight as a legitimate performing art by taking us into that world and sharing powerful moments in the nurse-patient relationship. For the very first time, the nursing profession was represented on stage as a talent in the Miss America Pageant. This act was a defining moment for nurses, and it created a reaction. A ripple effect began at that moment, and it wasn't all good.

I recognized her humility at once as she walked out to her mark plainly dressed in scrubs and sneakers with her stethoscope around her neck. She delivered her monolog with solemnity and compassion. In her description of the exchange with her patient, she demonstrated honest caring to Joe. He validated her role as a caregiver too when he declared that she was "HIS NURSE!" and that this was what mattered most to him. Her talent for this pageant was simply being a nurse. I believed she won the whole thing in that moment.

This act was moving to me as it must have been for many other nurses. I was proud to see a nurse performing as a nurse in a Miss America Pageant. I felt that nursing was for the first time recognized as a talent, a performance art, and this was going to bring to the forefront the special and extraordinary gifts nurses have. The non-tangible experience was a magical moment of connection. This effect is so hard to describe, measure, or artificially generate. This phenomenon cannot be taught in nursing school or ordered by a physician. Kelley's "Just a Nurse" story was sweet, honest, and filled with the enthusiasm a new nurse experiences as she continues to grow into her role.

No one could have foreseen the drama that would be played out in the days afterward. We saw the sacredness of Kelley's performance trifled and criticized by harsh comments on the popular daytime TV talk show *The View* the next day.

"She came in a nurse's uniform and basically read her emails out loud, and shockingly did not win," mocked one host.

"Why did she have a doctor's stethoscope around her neck?" another asked.

I don't need to rehash all the details. YouTube has several clips you can find if you want to get your blood pressure up a notch or two.

The comments struck some nerves as thousands of angered viewers responded. The internet blew up with outrage for the show's unfortunate mistake. Rumors of sponsors pulling advertising floated around as nurses across the country took social media by storm. Nurses pushed back loud and clear in solidarity for their profession, and the show took a smack in the chops for the error. The network did what they could to mend the situation, and the show hosts took a lot of heat for their comments.

The positive side to this is that nursing was brought forward and celebrated in ways never before seen in such a public way. The show in the crosshairs even rebounded with tribute segments for nurses and restated their support for nurses and the nursing profession at length in several opportunities following the initial insult. I hope this situation ended in forgiveness for all involved, but I also hope that nursing will have gained continued appreciation as a high art, as well as an honored and sacred profession.

As the TV hosts scrambled to undo the damage in the aftermath, the dialogue among working nurses across the country forever added the phrases "Not Just a Nurse" and "Doctor Stethoscope" to our remembrance of this nurse awakening. If America did not appreciate nursing as a talent before, it does now. Thank you, Kelley.

Nurses continuously list at the top of Gallup Poll's surveys, leading by 12% over the runners-up as the profession with the highest ethical standards in 2013. Nurses ranked as most trustworthy with 82% of Americans ranking their honesty as "very high" or "high." Runners up include pharmacists and grade school teachers tied at 70%, and doctors a close 3rd at 69%. [21]

With this newfound appreciation for the talent of being a nurse, I hope nurses everywhere will continue to realize the artistry of our profession. If for some of you the enthusiasm has faded or diminished over time, I'd like to offer some new tools to reinvigorate your passion for the work. The hopeful spirit of brand new nurses is a good place to reconnect with our calling and rediscover some of our earlier passion.

I experienced a significant boost in my love for nursing as I watched my oldest daughter graduate from the very same nursing school I attended 20 years earlier. A flood of memories from my glory days rushed over me, mixed with the intense pride of seeing my daughter join me in this noblest of professions. She and I now share a deeper understanding and connection with a language all our own. It is comforting to know I will have a nurse in the family to help make those hard decisions and provide a watchful eye over my care someday. When it's my time to check out and head to my big birthday bash in heaven, the nurse at my bedside will not be "just a nurse." I hope she will be wearing a clown nose and a smile for me.

PART III: METHOD

CHAPTER 13
THE CLINICAL ARTIST'S TOOLBOX

*"The artist is always beginning. Any
work of art which is not a beginning, an
invention, a discovery is of little worth."*

—Ezra Pound

I HOPE YOU HAVE FOUND SOMETHING useful in my personal story. Next, I will show you how and where I found the knowledge to become a clinical performer and share my best Magic Nurse secrets in Magic, Clowning, and Music so you may consider using these tools and resources for your own adventures into the arts. The gift of entertaining is much easier than you would imagine; it simply requires the desire to do it.

Everyone has their own unique perspective and can create their own performances. You may choose whatever item speaks to you and excites your imagination. Each trick in my magic toolbox has a specific purpose I appreciate for its high value as a useful distraction, a comfort, a therapeutic goal, or a memento of the caring performance experience. The mementos are just small gifts that remind the patient they were cared for and valued by their magic nurse.

There is no particular order to use these effects. I have plenty to choose from and use whatever fits each circumstance by being most suitable and beneficial to my patient and their family. As a clinician, you are best able to assess when to use these performance items to their best benefits.

The sources for education and networking are just as important as the items you can buy, if not more so. Be prepared to make new friends in the entertainment world. There are many professional and amateur performers within magic, clowning, and music organizations who will be eager to help you along the way. Entertainers with hearts of gold have been readily offering their talents to our medical world for many years. Magicians and clowns will become the most entertaining friends you will ever know. I have been personally blessed by those I have journeyed with, and could not be more thankful for the lifelong friendships forged in the arts.

CLOWN MAGIC

All the magic I do as a clinical magician works for clowns too. Though there are distinctive artistic differences between magicians and clowns, there are many places where these two art forms merge and share in each other's gifts. There are those, however, who cringe at the thought of blending these arts.

Magician purists would never think of putting a red nose on to do magic. I know magicians who really do not like clowns and prefer that clowns stay out of the magic business. I also know clowns whose magic ability is on par or superior to some working magic professionals.

There are also clown purists who would not dare mix magic with their performances. Usually these are professional circus clowns keeping to the traditions of visual and physical comedy only and often nonverbal. As with any theatrical profession, there are expectations for adhering to the art form. One would not expect to see river dancing at a ballet or a barbershop quartet at the opera.

The point I want to express here is that all the magic I perform whether as a clown character, clinical magician, or even as a regular nurse all work perfectly in the hospital, no matter what character I am playing. As a hospital clown, I believe everything is open to you, so bring whatever speaks to you…even magic!

TOOLS FOR CLINICAL MAGICIANS

D'Lite "Magic Lights from Anywhere!"

Available from any online magic store or directly from www.dlite.com. I recommend using a pair of the regular or ultra-bright red lights. These magic thumb tips allow you to manipulate a magic light on your fingertips, making it appear and disappear at your pleasure. As distraction, the game-play opportunities are limitless and can be a great routine for 15 seconds or 5 minutes. Perfect for patients with a pulse oximetry probe on their finger, where the clinical magician simply borrows the light from the patient to begin the routine.

Used for: distraction, performance.

Tricky Paddles "Rabbit in the Hat Paddle"

Available from any online magic store. This is pocket trick allows you to make a rabbit appear out of a hat not once but twice, then vanish both of them. It uses a simple sleight of hand method called the "paddle move," which you can master in minutes. It is not only a suburb magic effect that I use as a performance piece, but I also teach this trick as part of my therapeutic magic teaching.

Used for: performance, magic therapy, distraction.

Two Card Monte "A Game You Can't Lose"

As the name suggests, this is a card trick that uses only two cards. It is difficult to explain but easily learned when shown. The performer engages the spectator in a game where two cards are shown, one face up and the other face down in his/her hands. Then the face-up card is shown as it is placed behind the back. The other card remains face down. Asking the spectator to name the face down card, he is shocked to learn that they have switched places. This is repeated with the same surprising result. In the end, the cards have magically changed to have both faces on one card and both backs on the other.

I use this as a performance piece and teach it to patients as a therapeutic magic effect. I often give the two "magically changed" cards away as a memento of the magic encounter.

Used for: Performance, magic therapy, memento.

Svengali Deck "A Trick Deck that Does Magic All By Itself"

If you are of a certain age, you may have seen TV commercials for "TV Magic Cards" being performed by the famous magician Marshall Brodien. This was also a Svengali deck ideally suited for young magicians ages 8 and up, and these trick decks inspired the careers of many professional magicians working today. There are literally hundreds of card routines that can be performed with a Svengali deck. The best types use red or blue Bicycle decks and are found in any magic store. This effect is best for older kids, teenagers, and adults.

Used for: Performance only.

Rubber Band Magic "Hopping Rubber Bands"

Close-up magicians love being able to perform magic with common household items. Rubber band magic is a staple of any sleight of hand performer. Three simple variations are taught in Kevin Spencer's Healing of Magic program [12] that have great therapeutic value for patients to learn. Occupational therapists using this form of magic to help patients with flexion and extension of fingers also appreciate the motivational value and self-esteem of accomplishing this magic effect. Rubber band magic can also be found in David Copperfield's *Project Magic Handbook*. [11]

Used for: Performance, magic therapy, memento.

Napkin Roses "Twist a Napkin into a Memory"

Available from www.Napkinrose.com or any magic store. These come in packs of 50 or 150 in red, yellow, pink, white, and purple. I use these as a performance piece and frequently follow with a song on the ukulele. In hospital visits especially, I like to bring a dozen to give to the patients and teach them how to make them too. This great product, created by my friend and fellow magician Michael Mode, is one of the best effects in my repertoire.

Used for: Performance, magic therapy, distraction, comfort, memento.

Spring and Ring "A Mind-Bending Puzzle"

A staple in many commercial kid's magic sets, this simple metal puzzle designed for ages 8 and older is a real fooler. The spectator is shown a spring with a small ring locked in the coils and is asked to remove it. When unable to do so, the magician does it easily time and again. Often I reveal the secret after the routine and give the puzzle as a memento. This is a favorite item for those patients who wish to learn easy magic to perform for their caregivers and visitors. This can fool doctors too.

Used for: Performance, magic therapy, memento.

I regularly carry these items and a few others in my scrubs every day. These are enough to get you started on the road to becoming a great clinical magician. I have hundreds of other tricks I love using in this work, but I really prefer the ones I can teach and share with patients, staff, and families to empower them to discover magic of their own. If the magic bug is biting you, I would like to direct you to my favorite places to learn more.

MAGIC CLUBS AND NETWORKS

The best way to learn magic is from other magicians. When you visit a traditional magic store, there will usually be a skilled magician working behind the counter who can demonstrate tricks and help you select good magic effects for your purposes. This would also be a good person to ask about local magic clubs you can visit to make new magic friends and find mentors. I have been blessed by many great magician mentors, and now it is my turn to pass along a little bit of knowledge to others too.

Joining a magic club will be very helpful. When I found the Dallas Magic Club, I was pleased to find that there were other medical professionals among their ranks already. I became fast friends with several doctors who enjoy magic as a hobby and many who also use magic in their clinical settings. Magic clubs also offer special guest lectures by top magic professionals from around the world who perform and teach magic effects, principles, and skills to club members. Find a magic club through one of the sources below and your magic training will be on the fast track to success.

Society of American Magicians - S.A.M.

This is the oldest and most prestigious magical society in the world. Founded in 1902, the famous Harry Houdini was the society president from 1917 until his death October 31, 1926. You can learn more at their website www.magicsam.com. Local Magic clubs and chapters meet monthly and can be found in many major cities. I belong to the Dallas Magic Clubs (S.A.M. Assembly # 13 and I.B.M Ring # 174) found at: www.dallasmagic.org.

International Brotherhood of Magicians - I.B.M.

This is the world's largest magician organization with members in 88 countries, founded in 1922. More information can be found at: www.magician.org. Local branches, or "Rings," meet each month in hundreds of locations.

The Magic Cafe "Magicians Helping Magicians"

This forum website was founded in 2001 by Steve Brooks, producer, publisher, and magician. The Magic Cafe has over 62,000 members and nearly 5.5 million posts in a wide variety of magic topics. I found it to be a great resource for magic education, advice, and networking. Visit and join at www.themagiccafe.com.

MAGIC BOOKS, PUBLICATIONS, AND PROGRAMS

As an introduction to the many aspects of magic, *Mark Wilson's Complete Course in Magic* by Mark Wilson [22] has been favored most by professional and amateur magicians since 1975. Found in any magic store or online bookstore, it has over 2000 illustrations with precise step by step instructions. If I had to limit myself to one magic book only, this would be the one I'd pick.

David Copperfield's *Project Magic Handbook* is designed to combine selected magic effects with the arts of medicine to provide therapeutic activities for patients. [11]

Healing of Magic by Cindy and Kevin Spencer is a complete guide to building a therapeutic program in clinical settings. [12] Its manual and DVD describes how magicians and clinicians can work closely together to develop a defined magic program within the organization to offer magic activities as a hands-on occupational therapy program. Building on the concepts of Project Magic, Kevin and Cindy Spencer continue to make magic a more powerful tool in physical and occupational therapy settings. Program materials are ordered directly at www.magictherapy.com.

Side-FX: Clinically Relevant Magic Effects and Tricks for the Health-Care Provider by Scott Tokar and Harrison J. Carroll is well illustrated with effects using common props found in a typical physician's office. [23] Highly recommended for doctors, especially pediatricians.

Harlan Tarbell wrote *Tarbell Course in Magic* [10] for the serious magic student, and no magic library would be complete without this revered set of eight hardback books. First published in 1927 as a complete professional course, this set is now in its 14th printing and still favored among magic professionals. For clinical artists, I would not suggest this unless you plan on quitting your day job for a career in magic. I have it in my library, but I am not heading to Vegas anytime soon. Houdini had two personal sets.

For over 20 years Jeff McBride's Magic & Mystery School has educated magicians from around the world. Located in Las Vegas, the school offers several local and online classes. Of particular interest is the specialized Medicine and Magic Seminar for physicians, nurses, and therapists. Information can be found at www.magicalwisdom.com.

TOOLS FOR THE CLOWN DOCTOR

Developing your Performance Character

If you are a real doctor or nurse with courage and creativity, you are about to learn how you can bring a whole new level of joy you might only have dreamed about to your practice. You must be well established as a competent and reliable clinician before you take that sharp left turn into the clown world and find your inner "Patch Adams." Blending comedy and tragedy takes a true actor and you must be able to turn it on and off at the right times. Merging the clown and clinician into one person takes desire and good training.

You already have all that you need to be therapeutic in your assessment capabilities and actions. Behind your red nose is a trained medical mind with the ability to see the patient clearly and bring therapeutic value to your performance. The real power is the fact that with all your years of serious training and experience, you will put on a red nose and break down a barrier to connect on a completely different level. For therapeutic clowns to be truly therapeutic, it takes the ability to clinically assess and evaluate the outcomes for therapeutic patient goals. A clown doctor with medical assessment skills is a completely different kind of clown and will not be found in any circus. You have to learn comedy, throw out your stiff sense of self-importance, and become foolish!

The most important tools for the clown doctor are humor, comedic timing, improvisation, and acting. All of which can be learned if you do not already have natural talents for them. Equipped with these powers, you need only put on the red nose and a minimal costuming device that declares to the world you are a clown to be ready to play. You can even skip the nose if you have enough funny in you to become a silly character without it. Red Skelton is a great example of the ability to create a character by messing up his hair and making a few minor costume adjustments with a silly hat or glasses.

The most difficult hurdle to jump in becoming a clown doctor is giving yourself permission to play. Not only must you break all your own serious stereotypical behaviors to allow yourself to become a playful character, but you must also perform in an environment that will allow room and encouragement for such playfulness. Your fellow staff members and hospital administrators must also participate and join in, allowing for this exploration in clinical spaces. To be successful, agreement must be won for a more joyful and playful culture to be developed for the benefit of patient experiences. This might take considerable time to develop in some facilities, or it might happen quickly based on the readiness and desire to change the atmosphere and energy within a clinical environment. Desire for change is where it begins.

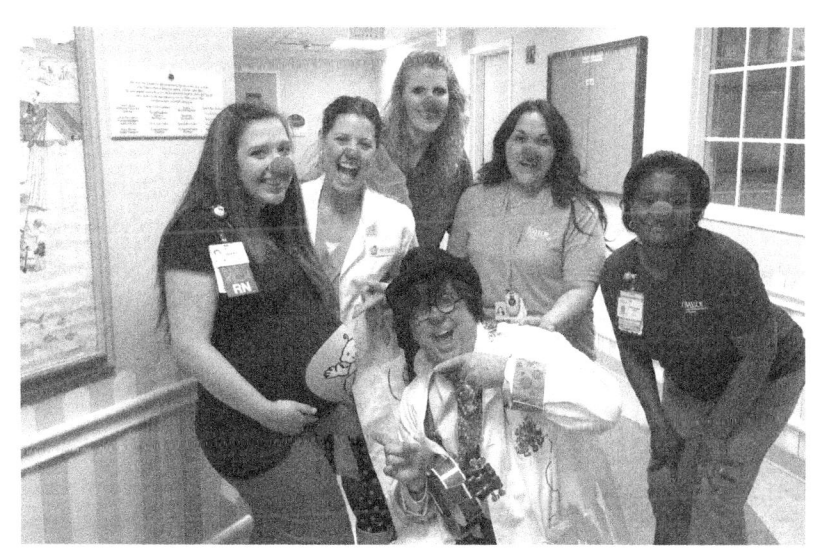

Rob Divers, RN

CLOWN SCHOOLS, TRAINING OPPORTUNITIES

New York Goofs

For premier theatrical clown training, Dick Monday and Tiffany Riley coordinate some of the best intensive clown training opportunities in the country. Joined by top performer/trainers in theater and circus, the Goofs have schools at various times throughout the year in New York and Dallas areas. To learn more about training visit their website at www.nygoofs.com.

Mooseburger Clown Arts Camp

This six-day intensive clown school located in Buffalo, Minnesota is designed to meet the needs of people who want to learn to be "real" working clowns. Since 1996, they teach all aspects of Clown Arts including hospital care clowning. Priscilla Mooseburger is an all-around source for everything that is clown as well as a premier designer for clown apparel. Tater's costumes were custom designed by Priscilla. Visit www.mooseburger.com for more information on the school and a wide variety of clowning supplies, performance props, and customized costume designs.

American Clown Academy

Offering a five-day camp teaching the fine art of clowning, this school is now in its fifth year. Started in 2012 by Jeff "Bungles the Clown" Potts and a cast of top clown instructors, it is growing each year. This school provides structured classes and one on one focus to help each clown develop their characters and routines. For more information, visit www.americanclownacademy.com.

CLOWN BOOKS, EDUCATION MATERIALS

A comprehensive study of clown history across the ages and diverse cultures, *Clowns* by John H. Towsen gives a solid foundation on the universal value of the clown in human experiences. [24] This was the first book I read to prepare me for clown school.

The Art of Clowning by Eli Simon on clown theory and character development is filled with exercises that develop performance skills. [25] If you cannot go to clown school, consider this a great home study course substitute.

The Moving Body by Jacques Lecoq is a classic treasure on theatrical techniques and improvisation explores movement gesture and expression. This is a high-level treatment of theatrical arts for serious students. [26]

Improv Wisdom by Patricia Ryan Madson will prepare you well for exploring the principles of improvisation for use in clinical comedy as well as in any other aspect of your life. By guiding you to learn and comprehend thirteen maxims of improvisation performance, you will find that improvisation is a natural choice for finding positive and exciting choices wherever you are. [27]

Clowning: Keep it Simple, Keep it Real by Angel Ocasio is a quick read to learn the key points of clowning arts. [28] I have had the great pleasure of learning from this great performer personally. If you can find him lecturing in a clown workshop or convention, he will show you how to be comfortable in your own clown skin. Find him at http://www.ocomedy.com/.

The Clown, from Heart to Heart by Ton Kurstjens, clown master and esteemed director in the Netherlands is a true inspiration for the clown artist to find within him/herself the heart of their clown and how to connect that loving intention to performances. To get this book, you must send an email to Ton directly: ton@clownerie.nl or visit his website and have Google/Bing translate the pages for you http://www.clownerie.nl/.

The Clown in You by Caroline Dream is a newer book published in 2014, and an essential work for both professional and beginner clowns. This is a deep dive into the mind of the clown and the core principles at work in this theatrical art form. Each master of this craft finds unique ways to guide us through the depths of this art form, paving new roads to journey upon as we discover our proper places behind the red nose. [29]

CLOWN ALLEYS AND MEMBERSHIP ORGANIZATIONS

Clowns of America International, COAI

This is the largest clown membership organization in North America and has alley members all around the world. This great organization publishes a fantastic bi-monthly magazine called *The New Calliope* filled with resources for professional clowns and clown artists of all ages and experience levels. National conventions are held annually around the country. I belong to the Dallas COAI chapter, Texas Mid-Cities Clown Alley #85. Visit www.COAI.org for more information.

Texas Clown Association, TCA

Many states have locally organized groups, but Texas is among those that have a robust clown organization for professional and volunteer clowns to learn the craft. State conventions provide extensive learning opportunities and networking. Visit www.texasclownassociation.org.

CLOWN HUMANITARIAN AND RELIEF ORGANIZATIONS

Red Nose Response, RNR

Founded in 2005 to unite the clown community for support relief operations, this North America based relief group provides volunteer clown responders to assist in the healing process following major natural or man-made catastrophes. Educational programs and disaster preparedness presentations are also delivered with clown humor for kids and families to help educate about disasters without invoking fear. This group is close to my heart, and I serve on the board of this nonprofit organization with over 1000 registered volunteer clown responders. I strongly urge clowns with medical backgrounds to join this group. Visit www.rednoseresponse.org.

Gesundheit Institute

Founded by Patch Adams, MD in 1971, the Gesundheit Institute is a nonprofit healthcare organization with global reach. Devoted to changing America's healthcare system with the belief that laughter, joy, and creativity are an integral part of the healing process, the Gesundheit Institute supports several programs to teach and inspire caregivers around the world. In 2006, Gesundheit Global Outreach, GGO was formed to encompass humanitarian clowning missions and aid, educational programs, building projects, and community development around the world. Mission opportunities are open to anyone desiring to take their clowning seriously enough to make a difference in distressed and suffering communities. Visit www.patchadams.org.

The Dream Doctors Project: Medical Clowning in Action

This amazing program was started in 2002 and integrates medical clowns or "Dream Doctors" in hospitals throughout Israel. They have numerous published studies and articles regarding medical clowning. I believe this is the best source for information to develop this specialized form of clowning in clinical spaces. Look into the research they have shared with the world at their website www.dreamddoctors.org.il/en/.

"I Clown You" Documentary

The "I Clown You" Documentary is currently filming and will soon release a comprehensive exposition of the excellent medical clown work being done in Israel. The expansion of creative arts in medicine is clearly a cutting-edge technology in the most human way. Love is the active ingredient for medical clowns. Learn more at http://www.

iclownyoudoc.com/ and https://www.facebook.com/IClownYou

Clowns Without Borders, CWB

This amazing worldwide humanitarian clown effort has organizations in twelve countries with ongoing missions and projects in distressed communities everywhere. CWB-USA was formed in 1995 and continues to run as a robust volunteer-run organization providing much-needed laughter and humor to children and persons in areas of crisis. Visit their website at: www.clownswithoutborders.org.

A WORD ON CLOWN PROPS

In the world of a clown, there are no limits to the comedic value of any object, real or imagined. The clown brain discovers the joy in the world and draws out the funny through improvisation technique from everything in reach. It is perspective—a way of seeing the world—which makes anything a usable prop for a clown bit, skit, or performance piece. This learned ability will serve you better than any commercial prop, gag, or device you can buy.

There are however many funny props that are favored among clowns, and I could not resist adding some of them in my clowning. My favorite props are those that allow others to join me in my clown world and play along. Engaging and connecting with the patients, staff, and anyone in my path by sharing in a fun and unexpected activity brings out the most favorable responses I have experienced. I especially like to "deputize" all those who, for a moment, wish to become a clown with me and let their repressed clown energy out for a bit.

This magically happens when you give your newfound clown friend a red nose to wear. I have a never-ending supply of sponge clown noses I give away. It's not fair that I get to be silly and not them. By placing a clown nose on them, we have just equalized the game and can play together. The silliness that happens next is whatever naturally develops in that moment. I am continually surprised by the games that emerge and the funny that occurs in these completely natural moments.

Once the red noses are in place, there are any number of playful props you can employ to play games with. Some of the items are best for workshop or group settings where I can help kids learn new physical skills with a clowning theme. Other items are best for strolling in hospital settings as a performance piece.

Sponge Clown Noses

Goshman Foam Clown Noses Created by Magic by Gosh, Inc. are the best quality product for hospital use in my opinion. Gosh is a legendary name in the world of magic due to the fact that every magician who does sponge ball magic is likely using Gosh sponge balls. There are several sources available for noses on the internet and from hospital clown specific websites also.

Steve Goshman is a wonderfully funny and talented man who took special care to produce a sponge nose product of the highest quality that would be suitable for patients. These noses are colorfast and do not run or bleed onto the skin. Available in red, green, and pink, the colors are fused into the sponge material and not dyed like many other lower quality noses.

Goshman sponge products have a much softer feel and are gentler on sensitive skin. Steve and I became friends in 2015, and he has such love for clowns and others who focus their talents on helping kids who need it most. You can find these great noses at www.hospitalclown.com or www.clownantics.com and many other online clown and magic stores. If you need a large order for hospital or other nonprofit work, contact me directly and I will help facilitate your order.

World's Largest Underpants

This novelty prop sports an endless amount of fun because there is a great amount of comedy value in underwear. I can't explain why this works, but it just does. I call it the "nuclear option" when I whip out the big drawers to get the party started. This is a powerful visual prop that generates a large amount of funny. You can even get a few of your friends to climb inside for a pseudo sack race or to parade around, tossing modesty and dignity to the wind. These can be found at multiple online sources. I purchase my plus size skivvies from Archie McPhee. www.mcphee.com.

Farts are Funny

Any prop you can find that delivers this performance piece (other than the usual biological method) will bring laughs in any language around the world. The best are amplified electronic devices or phone applications for delivering the goods in the widest variety of sounds and realistic characteristics. With the motion sensors in smartphones, some apps can be motion activated to squeak off a sound. The iPhone has an app for fart noises that works by lifting your leg with the phone in your pocket. When this is amplified over a speaker, it is music to my ears! Check your iPhone App Store or Android Store and choose an app that meets your needs.

For you low tech folks, the original Whoopee Cushion is still a favorite though not suitable in latex free settings. As with anything, a simple Google/Bing search will provide ample suppliers.

Juggling Scarves

Juggling Scarves are brightly colored sheer nylon squares that float and fall gently for a slow, easy cascade. Often used for teaching the concepts of juggling, these are favored for their portability and ease of use. Available in neon colors, pink, blue, and yellow, they bring a beautiful display of color and fun to an otherwise bland clinical setting. I use these to empower patients by teaching them how to pass-juggle with me. Within seconds, I have had many patients juggling with me to festive music, much to their own amazement.

Aside from juggling, these are a wonderful implement to use in improvisation or as a costuming accessory that is also valuable for play therapy. I personally use juggling scarves from: www.dube.com, an online web store for jugglers. Another popular source for juggling supplies is www.renegadejuggling.com. Both companies have everything under the sun in juggling and other circus performance props.

Clown Noise Makers

I could not possibly list all the gems I have seen from other hospital clowns and performers of all types that are great for entertaining patients of all ages. Creating sounds that fill the space with happiness can be delivered in countless ways. Such items as kazoos, penny whistles, recorders, flutes, tambourines, bells, whistles, rattles, squeakers, clappers, xylophones, juice harps, and the list goes on. Find your own inspiration for making joyful noise and use it. Any musical instrument can be used if it fits the user and produces the desired results. Even a can of Spam can join your act as a "one string wonder" called the Spamjo (canjo). I'm not kidding! Visit www.spamjo.com and see for yourself.

Portable Sound Systems

No matter what kind of character you create for your clinical performances, you should try to add some sort of music accompaniment. If you like to sing, you should try to find ways to bring this gift with you also. It can be silly or beautiful; it is entirely up to you. You could bring a portable MP3 player for any number of recorded music tracks or silly sound effects. I personally use my smartphone and a Bluetooth portable speaker when I want to make clown rounds with mood music. There are so many good options to choose from in selecting your own recordings. The Hokey Pokey is still a classic. This is your show, so create a soundtrack that best suits you.

Singers and Vocalists

Singing is an essential tool in clown work. It does not matter if you sing well or not; it is a performance skill you can use everywhere. A sweet or funny song or sing-a-longs work great. I sang TV theme songs to kids during PICC line placements as a distraction that negated the need for sedation. Gilligan's Island, The Brady Bunch, and Beverly Hillbillies theme songs are my favorites. Often parents would join in on the nostalgia and sing along too. Working as a sedation nurse, I often tried to offer the non-pharmaceutical option of being entertaining to win cooperation and trust for those procedures where we sedated for fear and anxiety alone. Short duration diagnostic imaging studies were always my favorite time to help kids find their own super powers and avoid sedation drugs.

Barbershop Harmony

If you are a pretty good singer or have ever been in a school or church choir, take special note of what I am about to tell you. The soothing chords of four-part harmony are a wonderful sound to experience, and there are wonderful places to improve your talents and find new ways to enjoy vocal music. Explore a great American vocal music art called Barbershop.

I joined the Barbershop Harmony Society and perform with the Vocal Majority Chorus based in Dallas, TX. Visit www.vocalmajority.com or search YouTube for Vocal Majority to see what I am talking about. If you have not yet discovered the world of barbershop harmony, you are missing out on the best opportunities I know of to express and develop your vocal talents.

For ladies, the sister organization is known as the Sweet Adelines International.

Both organizations have local chapters with choruses everywhere and are nonprofit with similar missions to use four-part a-Capella singing to spread the joy of harmony to a troubled world. This musical society and art form will give you vocal training and increased confidence as an overall show performer. Check out these great organizations and find a local chapter to visit and join if you wish to make vocal music one of your super powers: Barbershop Harmony Society, BHS at www.barbershop.org and Sweet Adelines International at www.sweetadelines.com

YOUR MUSICAL TOOLBOX

In the entertainment world, there is no end to the possibilities you can adapt for your practice. The most important performance tools are those that bring you the most personal enjoyment when you use them. You cannot get the desired effect for a patient if it does not first have the same effect on you. For art to be healing, it has also to be healing to ourselves in the process of developing it, and again as we share it with others. This is a key component to the nature of bidirectional care. If you take the time to learn a difficult or complex performance art, it will be life changing for you. When you then bring this to work, you are helping yourself and others in a much more connected way. Medical professionalism maintains a certain barrier from our patients, but art crosses over and delivers something special, intangible, and more valuable than a medical treatment. I implore you to become an explorer in your own creative life and find those performance tools that are best for you.

MUSICAL INSTRUMENTS

Singing a song is nice, but an instrument to accompany vocals adds a whole new layer to the performance. The ideal instrument is obviously one that you can play well, but size and portability are a factor too. Learning any instrument can be challenging, even the ones that are considered "easy to learn." It will take time, so relax and take all the time you need. When you can play a handful of songs that you are going to sing, you will really enjoy having these gifts to share.

In this next section I will focus on the three instruments I like best for hospital work, which are the ukulele, harmonica, and concertina, though any musical instrument ever invented will work if you love it enough!

The Ukulele

My personal favorite is the ukulele. I believe it is the easiest of the three to learn and best for accompanying a singing voice. The guitar is also great, but I downsized to the ukulele for ease of use.

Ukuleles come in various sizes: soprano, concert, tenor, and baritone (from smallest to largest). It is best to go with the smallest size where your fingers can move easily upon the fretboard without tripping over each other. The concert size was best for my hospital clown character, but I soon stepped up to the tenor size for Tater's stage performances and my ElfVis character that I use for special events.

Beginning at around thirty bucks, you will find that once you get your feet wet with this instrument, you might acquire several more before long. I have five ukuleles total and am trying my best to resist getting just one more. There are many brands that are really good at very reasonable prices.

Find one that feels good in your hands and looks good to your eye. Guitar Center has a good selection, as do many good music stores that carry stringed instruments. You can also purchase online, though it is hard to fall in love with an instrument you haven't held in your hands. Feeling how the fret board feels under your fingertips is helpful to see if the size is right for you. Tonal quality is another aspect I like to hear in person, moving from one uke to another in the selection process at the music store is a ritual I prefer when picking out a good ukulele. Once you start learning how to play chords, you will see why this is important. For a good quality instrument, you can expect to pay between $200 and $300 for a ukulele you could perform professionally with. Prices start to climb much higher for the best quality instruments played by top musicians and recording artists.

Most ukuleles are made from wood, but they don't have to be. Composite materials are also used in some designs, and there is one in particular I really like, made by a small company in Bend, Oregon called Outdoor Ukulele. Made from translucent polycarbonate, this instrument can withstand extreme temperatures and rugged outdoor conditions. Though you might not ever need to visit the Antarctica or the rim of an active volcano, this ukulele will play nicely whether it's

-40 or 250 degrees outside. These can take a beating and be completely cleaned with hospital grade disinfectants. Visit: www.outdoorukulele.com to learn more.

Ukulele Resources Online

There are many online resources for just about anything you wish to learn. The best place to start is Google/Bing and YouTube. There are tutorials for just about everything posted by other enthusiasts. I have two favorite websites I use to keep my instrument tuned and learn new songs.

Doctor Uke: http://www.doctoruke.com/

The free songs and arrangements provided by Dr. Uke are the best I have found on the internet for learning great songs on the ukulele. There are over 1500 songs listed with lyrics and chord charts. Did I mention it was free? There are even streaming audio files accompanying most songs played and sung by the doctor himself! Nearly every song I perform today, I learned from Dr. Uke's website. But there is more, he happens to be a real doctor! Jim Rosokoff, MD is a retired dermatologist and manages the best free online ukulele music website on the internet. Dr. Uke and his two beautifully talented daughters perform together locally and in New York City as "Dr. Uke and Daughters" with a fantastic blend of vocal harmony.

Dr. Rosokoff also leads The Glastonbury Ukulele Band and promotes a robust ukulele club with members throughout Connecticut. I highly recommend this resource and Dr. Uke's club if you happen to be traveling near Glastonbury.

Online Ukulele Tuner:
www.get-tuned.com/online_ukulele_tuner.php

Though having a regular electronic tuner in your ukulele case is preferred, I have often just used this online website to tune up while at the computer before I head off to a gig.

Smartphone Ukulele Tuners

There are several applications available for Android and iPhones.

Rob Divers, RN

The Harmonica

This well-known pocket free reed instrument also called a French harp is great for bringing portable melodies anywhere. Though it's often used in blues music, it can be a cheerful sound to chase the blues away. I am not a harmonica player myself, but friends who use this instrument swear by it as a great tool for hospital work. Respiratory therapists have even discovered that this instrument is perfect for therapeutic uses with patients who have COPD and other pulmonary conditions. The actions of blowing and drawing air through a harmonica improve lung function. Learning a song on the harmonica has to be much more enjoyable for patients than sucking on an Incentive Spirometer. Once again, art meets medicine in a surprisingly wonderful way.

As with any musical instrument, price ranges vary on quality and maker from the tiniest four-hole version for about $4 to $25,000 for a Bob Dylan hand signed seven-piece harmonica set. You can jump in at whatever price point fits you. The Hohner is commonly known by many, but the serious harp enthusiast is aware of several other instruments made by highly rated makers such as Suzuki, Seydel, Lee Oscar, Johnson, Lumsing, and Swan. There are too many sources to list for more information on the harmonica. If this speaks to you, you know where to look.

The Concertina

The concertina is very similar to the accordion as it has buttons and a bellows, but is considerably smaller and lighter for strolling. This instrument may not be well-known today as popularity has declined considerably in modern time. The concertina has its origins in Germany and England in the early 1800s, and is still quite popular in folk music, especially in Europe. This unique looking instrument is widely available from music stores and online sources. Many are made by the same makers of fine harmonicas. Prices start below $200 for an entry level quality instrument.

Any musical instrument takes a considerable amount of time and practice to learn, but the rewards are always there waiting for you. The concertina is no different. You do have the ability to sing as you play along, and dancing is always a possibility when someone breaks out a concertina. The bright sounds and nostalgic appearance combine to add a dimensional quality to your performance character.

If you are a healthcare provider looking for renewed inspiration in your work, I pray you have found something to take away from this book. A single magic trick shared with a patient can begin your creative journey.

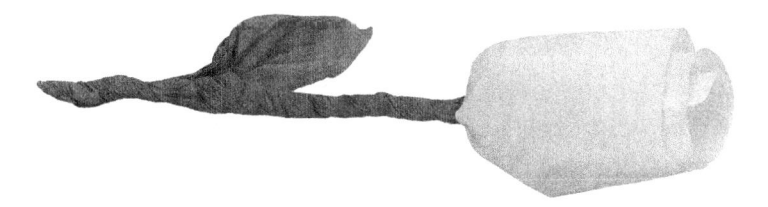

CHAPTER 14
INTEGRATING ART IN HOSPITAL SYSTEMS

> *"If care is to be the core of a health care system, then we care-givers need to re-think our abilities to respond to the variety of situations that the 21st century places us. We would like to see ourselves as a positive force towards changing the system as we want it to be, not just benchwarmers for the health care system as it is."*
>
> —Susan Parenti, DMA, Redesigning the Character of the Care-actor

WE HAVE THE BEST DISEASE care system in the world. Advances in IT and EHRs (electronic health records) are eclipsing human creativity. Diagnostic equipment performs scientific wonders, but the art of good bedside manner has disappeared to make room for data entry and medical clerking. This growth in technology has stolen the time and focus of medical professionals away from their patients. The clinician's eyes are fixed on computer screens in today's medical interview instead of seeing the hopes and fears present in the eyes of our patients. We have adjusted to the modern system with less care at the bedside. I believe we are in danger of losing the understanding of what "care" means in healthcare.

How much time, money, and effort go into recruitment and retention of staff? How many programs, training systems, and screening tools are used to select ideal employees to hire? How great would it be to develop the desired qualities in employees you already have, by encouraging the creativity that makes us better humans overall?

Staffing challenges persist due to increasing demand and shortages of nursing and other medical professionals. Not a week goes by where a new nursing job with a large sign on bonus doesn't show up in my mailbox. With an excellent offer of money and the promise of a better career knocking on my door, it would be easy to vacate one position to take another if I didn't feel a creative, artistic, personal sense of purpose in my current job. I have to think that if the culture of a hospital were healthy, loving, positive, and creative, staff retention and recruitment would be easier and less expensive.

Inspiring artistic growth in others fuels the imagination to break new ground. With compassionate intent fused with creativity, I experience a higher sense of purpose and effectiveness in my nursing practice. If you can imagine the possibilities from tapping into the creative talents of medical and nursing staff within your hospital, you can build a culture centered in creative compassion that strengthens the health of your organization and enhances the bedside manner your customers experience. There are many sleeping artists waiting for the invitation to blossom and grow instead of seeking new workplaces.

Stress is a constant underlying side-effect in this field, though we are conditioned to function as professionals and appropriately handle whatever happens. Many jobs are stressful, but the healthcare worker has the burden of participating in the personal tragedies of our fellow human beings every day. Nurses feel pain too. We are empathetic to their circumstances and shoulder the responsibility of disease treatment with stoic professionalism as we bounce from one patient to another for 12-hour shifts. Nurses have to develop a means within themselves to cope emotionally with the suffering and death they see. Burnout is a real problem for critical care nurses especially. ICU and ER nurses are the hardest positions to keep filled in hospitals everywhere. We have to find better ways to care for the caregivers if we desire our healthcare system to work better for the rest of us.

The powers of creative expression are the least used but most effective coping skills a burned-out nurse could have to self-treat for the harmful effects of hospital stress.

We need to take everyone's stress level down a few notches and create safe ways to reconnect with each other as a community within our hospital walls, rather than the technological nightmare we are building to deliver efficient goods and services while avoiding litigation. We can include a creative opportunity to integrate arts and humanities into our medical delivery systems, and it would help all of us in the long run.

Through magic and the red nose, I have found an immediate intervention that turns a nurse or doctor's day around. Using artistic tools provides opportunities to reconnect with our human emotions in a positive way, and this works for staff as well as for patients. If we can see the value in exploring a new way of treating our healthcare environments for both staff and patients, we can do more to heal our healthcare system than we may realize.

A hospital where a sense of community is encouraged and the artistic expression and uniqueness of each individual's personal contributions have value could attract and retain talented practitioners.

Performing art improves loving and compassionate caregiving and inspires staff to go the extra mile at a patient's bedside. Creating clinical performers empowered to connect with their patients, to make them smile, laugh, or share in a magic moment by performing a small act of kindness, develops immeasurable qualities that can make a powerful difference in the experience of patients and families.

While integrating ER software solutions at Emergisoft, Inc., I visited over thirty client hospital systems across the country as a Clinical Process Director. I witnessed multiple sites requiring unnatural scripting language of staff for the purpose of improving the customer experience. In fact, one of my responsibilities was to create, edit, and update the scripted medical language used in our physician documentation software to ensure revenue capture. When a doctor checks a box, my scripted medical language output creates the medical record in the EHR. Scripting is an effective way of controlling dialogue for consistency of message in a system, but the individuals using the script were not speaking for themselves in the patient interaction. The system was talking to the patient, diminishing their experience instead of improving it.

The use of customer service scripting might be okay for a department store chain at the mall, but it never comes across as genuine. By the very nature of why a patient requires healthcare, genuine compassion has to be present for them to trust and cooperate with the healthcare provider. When I hear a nurse using a phrase, "I am raising your side rails to ensure your safety," it sounds forced. "I am drawing closed your curtain for your privacy." I do not hear genuine care about privacy. When they eventually get the survey that asks those specific questions about safety and privacy, they are supposed to remember you specifically addressed those for their benefit. However, I believe a disproportionate number of surveys are filled out by unhappy people who had too many scripted experiences and not enough real ones.

Every individual caregiver and patient are different, and any combination of the two will result in a unique interaction that leaves a lasting impression on both. Rather than using scripts and stilted language, we would be better served teaching our staff to become better improvisational "care-actors" with improved ability to think on the fly as improvisation artists who drive positive outcomes with their creative talents, wit, and compassion.

If we could do more to stand out in more unique and genuine ways, we might leave a memorable impression in the minds of our patients and capture more positive surveys from those who otherwise would not have been motivated to return a survey response at all. We need happier customers who are getting something special from us.

Rob Divers, RN

Magnet Status is a high measure of excellence in a hospital organization and creates an environment where great nurses can grow and enhance excellent nursing practice. I think this would be the perfect place to include artistic creativity as well. There might be substantial value to bringing an Artistic Clinical Director into the organization to develop creative culture change based on the artistic application of therapeutic performing arts. A nurse who includes creativity in their craft will become an incredible asset because that caregiver is trained to be a compassionate care artist. That just sounds way cool to me. Having a few of these specialized practitioners in your hospital can go a very long way to enhance the organization and the community.

I've met talented consultants who specialize in process change management, helping clients create improved cultures and customer experience delivery systems. Customer survey results are key indicators of the performance of a hospital to the degree that many organizations spend valuable resources training their employees to be better customer service providers. I agree that improvements are often needed, but there is a more organic and natural way to inspire the entire culture of our workplace using personal creativity.

When I started doing magic at the bedside, it was just an act of kindness. It was not in my job description, but I considered it a personal mission to go the extra mile. The momentum to explore magic in my practice continued. When I began using magic as a therapy by teaching tricks to empower patients, the results were so compelling. It completely changed the direction of my clinical career.

Finding the personal value of using magic and improvisational comedy in my hospital work has been a continuous process of discovery of creating meaningful and positive experiences in my patient interactions. Over and again, people refer to the name Patch Adams when thanking me for doing something fun with them. It is a descriptive way of putting a label on a particular behavior universally appreciated in a medical setting. The Patch Adams movie has set a standard of care that people recognize when they see it. Establishing a genuine connection conveys care better than anything I know, and we can re-learn this lost art of medicine. There is something to this "Patch" idea.

Since 1999 I have thought about how clinical performance art could be practical and safe in hospital systems without interfering with the complex organizational structures that minimize risks, maintain high standards, and treat patients with the highest medical care possible.

Professional and environmental cultures and departmental variables also present challenges, as each specialty area also has sub-culture and unique issues to consider for each clinical space. Calling upon all my experiences clinically and creatively, I would like to share a simple blueprint for designing a program for the talented clinical artists in your hospital organization. Creativity only needs a tiny protected space to make an impact on an organization. I am hopeful more leaders in healthcare will be inspired to provide similar concepts that incorporate performance driven enhancements by individual caregivers with specialized training to achieve desired outcomes.

It begins by creating a performance team to lead the way for the hospital. Designing a sustained program will provide the framework to allow for creative exploration of activities for the organization. Through support and encouragement of artistic performance, allowing trained clinical performing artists to find opportunities and areas we can nurture creative change throughout the hospital. Small acts of creative art can provide a medium for a healthy culture to develop naturally. We must allow our best clinical actors the freedom and encouragement to express creativity in their roles.

Establishing a new culture where this exploration of music, comedy, magic, and other therapeutic performances are fused with clinical competence makes the highest levels of patient and job satisfaction possible. By creating the opportunity for a performance team, the most motivated and talented staff will consider it a privilege and honor to volunteer and donate back their time and talents for the chance to perform as therapeutic performing artists.

I believe you can design and launch a clinical arts program in any hospital that can inspire revolutionary change for a more positive and creative culture throughout the organization.

If you build it, they will come.

Here is a simple outline of the steps to create a program within your hospital. The level of support and the encouragement of talent within the organization will be necessary to consider in each case. The opportunity is there. The precedent has already proved successful in hospitals around the world that have developed medical clown programs. I think we can build on the success of the pioneers in the medical clown profession, by inviting medical talent to participate. All that is needed is the desire and commitment for creating something new.

Clinical Performing Arts Program
- Form a committee to design the operative policies and goals of the program.
- Establish key leadership roles to administrate the Performing Arts Team.
- Create an Artistic Clinical Director position to guide the program.
- Partner with the arts organizations in your community to bring as much outside talent as possible to share in this creative mission to benefit your patients and staff.
- Involve media relations, volunteer services, Chaplain, other affected departments.
- Design the size and makeup of your performing team at 4 to 8 members, possibly more.
- Hold hospital-wide auditions to select candidates from interested doctors, licensed clinicians, and other skilled medical staff.
- Bring your talent pool to professional levels through artistic instruction from established programs.

- Provide continuing educational opportunities to train interested staff in clowning, magic, music, and theatrical or performance art from established programs.
- Provide internal workshops open to all staff members to share in the growth process of artistic expression. Sponsor hospital-wide talent shows for culture enhancement.
- Provide media relations with the opportunity to promote your artistic programs and events to the community.

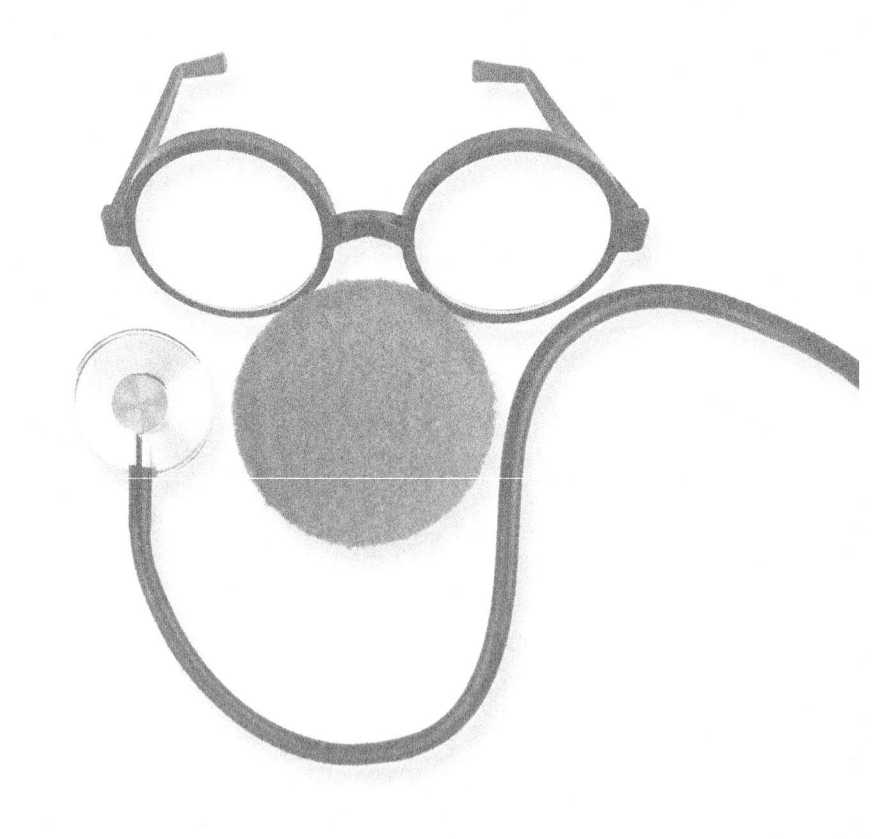

ACKNOWLEDGEMENTS

My mother, Judith Diane Divers, never doubted me when, on any given day, I declared I was an astronaut, mind reader, magician, scientist, ventriloquist, or Spiderman. The wild imaginations and dreams of a child are the clay our moms use to create great human vessels of their children. Molding them by providing their imaginations with the tools necessary to explore: blanket forts, cardboard spaceships, tinfoil helmets, wrapping tube swords, or phasers set on stun.

Patch often says, "Everything good in me came from my mother!" The world owes an enormous debt of gratitude to Anna for cultivating the artist and healer in her son Hunter "Patch" Adams.

This book is a work of gratitude in honor of my mom, of course, but also to Brett's mother Karen, Kevin's mom Judy, Michael's mother Rose, and all moms who use their magic to inspire artists within their sons and daughters. In a hostile world, I believe the greatest power a mother has is the ability to wrap an indestructible force field of creative light around their children to protect their dreams and ward off evil.

As I reflected on my childhood, I had hardly noticed that my mother lived during the cold war with Russia where instant vaporization from a nuclear holocaust loomed in her reality. The carnage of Vietnam was shielded from view as I learned poetry, puppetry, and music. She intervened with executive pardon when Dad got too enthusiastic with his belt. I was protected to dream, imagine, love, and explore because a mother's barrier of love surrounded me. Racial tensions were set aside at a turbulent time when forced integration of segregated schools was carefully nurtured by both black and white mothers hoping for the promised future of peaceful equality for their children. The 60s and 70s in South Florida had many problems to work out.

Today's dangers are no different, though today's mothers are stronger than ever before. Do not let evil outshine the good you desire. If we are going to survive as a species, it will be because the power of motherhood held her ground.

Mothers, teach your children well. The new world will need the best you can make.

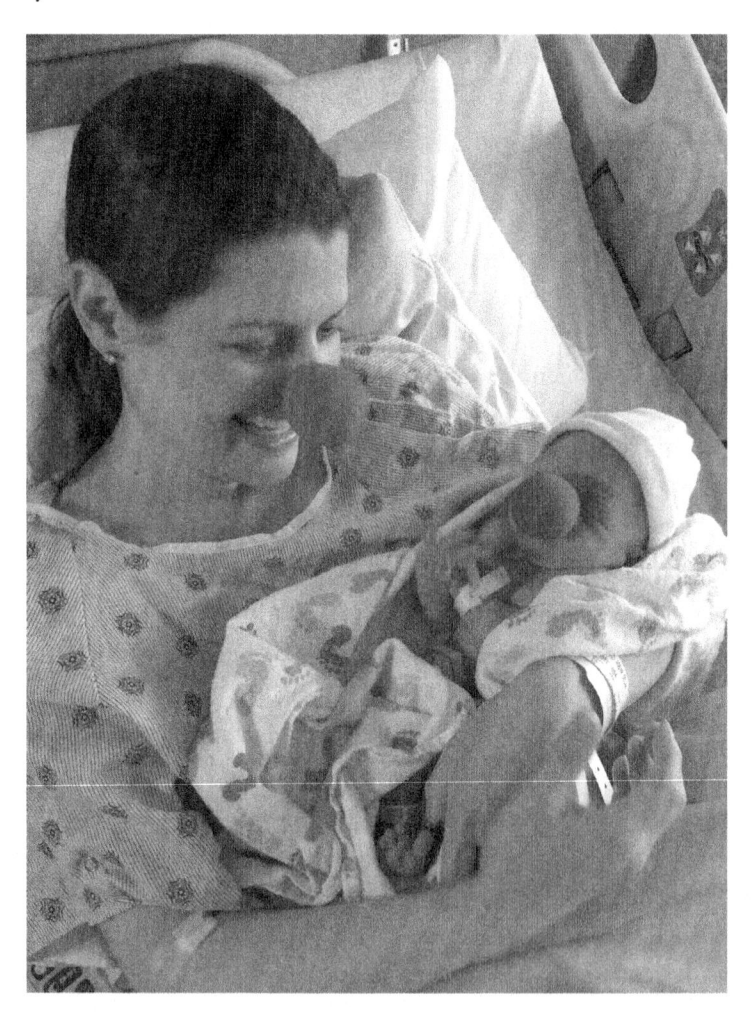

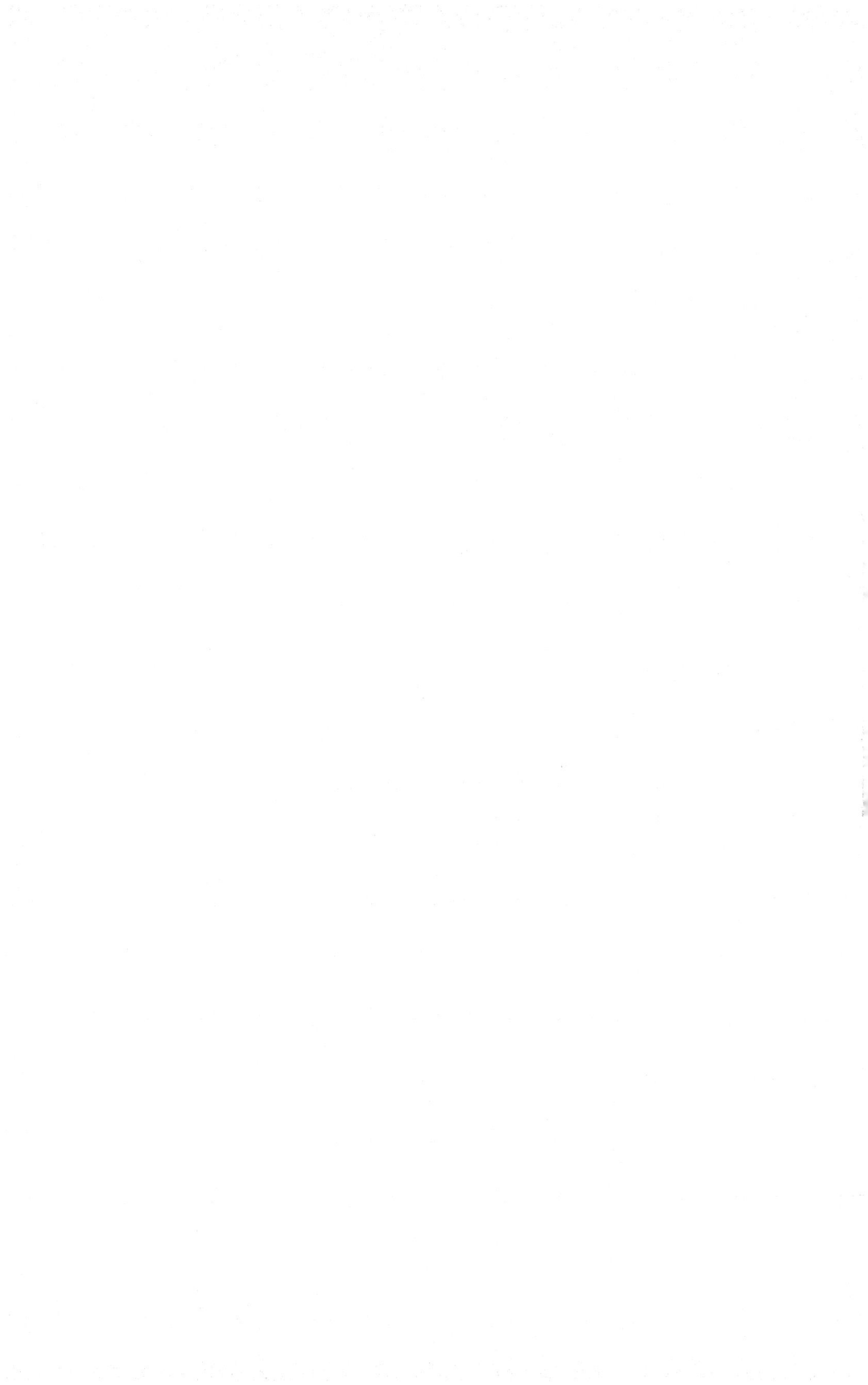

ABOUT THE AUTHOR

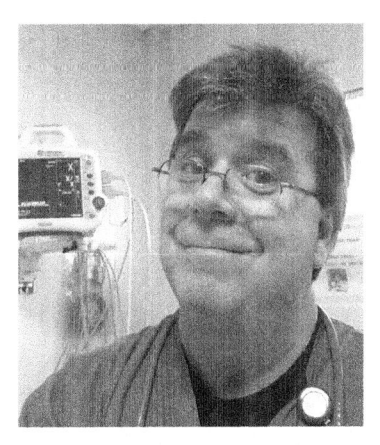

Rob Divers, RN graduated from Tarrant County College in 1994 and has been nursing for 23 years. Rob was certified in pediatric and adult trauma (ENPC and TNCC) and worked in the Emergency Room for 10 years prior to becoming specialized in pediatrics. While working in two major pediatric hospitals in the Dallas Area, he made it his mission to bring more joy into the lives of his patients through the use of well-timed, age appropriate comedy and magic. Magic Nurse, LLC was organized in 2012 to explore the use of creative arts in clinical practice and advance therapeutic magic and medical clowning for medical professionals.

With a lifelong passion for music, Rob performs around the country with the Vocal Majority Chorus and is a member of the Barbershop Harmony Society. He regularly volunteers as a camp nurse for the Spina Bifida Association of North Texas and makes hospital visits as a medical clown and clinical magician for adult and pediatric patients in the Dallas/Ft. Worth area.

Rob is a Texas Scottish Rite Mason and a member of the Society of American Magicians, Texas Association of Magicians, Clowns of America International, and Texas Clown Association, and recently received lifetime recognition as a DFW Great 100 Nurse for 2017

REFERENCES

1. US Department of Labor. "Occupational employment projections to 2016". https://www.bls.gov/opub/mlr/2007/11/art5full.pdf
2. Health Resources and Services Administration. "The US Nursing Workforce: Trends in Supply and Education". Am Nurs Today. 2014;9(6).
3. https://www.childrens.com/patient-resources/visitor-patient-guide/activities-for-kids/funnyatrics-clown-program and https://give.childrens.com/latest-news/latest-news-entry/childrens-health-funnyatrics-clown-program-turns-10
4. Kelly, Emmett, R Beverly Kelley. *Clown*. Buccaneer Books. Reprint Ed (May 1, 1996). https://www.amazon.com/Clown-Emmett-Kelly/dp/0899668127/
5. Learn more about Red Skelton's Freddy the Freeloader here http://red-skelton.info/articles/freddy-the-freeloader-red-skeltons-famous-hobo-clown/
6. Learn more about Glenn Beck's TV show *The Blaze* here http://www.theblaze.com/
7. Learn more about the School for Designing a Society project here http://www.designingasociety.net/
8. https://www.facebook.com/HOSPISONRISASCR
9. John Northern Hilliard. *Greater Magic: A Practical Treatise on Modern Magic*. Carl Waring Jones, privately printed for professional & amateur magicians. 1st Ed (1938). https://www.amazon.com/dp/B0007HGBEA/

10. Harlan Tarbell. *Tarbell Course in Magic Volume 1 thru 8*. D Robbins & Co, Inc. 14th Printing (1996). https://www.amazon.com/D-Robbins-Tarbell-Course-Magic/dp/B002YNCWXE
11. Organized in 1981 by David Copperfield and Julie DeJean, O.T.R. Concept and program created by David Copperfield. Written by Richard Kaufman. Illustrated by Earle Oakes. *David Copperfield's Project Magic Handbook*. (2002) https://www.amazon.com/Copperfields-Project-Handbook-Concept-Copperfield/dp/B002518NG0/
12. Spencer, Kevin and Cindy Spencer. *Healing of Magic*. Spencer Productions. Second Ed (1999). http://www.magictherapy.com/
13. Learn more about Kevin Spencer's curriculum in Hocus Focus http://www.hocusfocuseducation.com/hocus-focus/introduction-to-hocus-focus/
14. http://projectmagic.org/
15. http://www.circusesandsideshows.com/circuses/bigapplecircus.html
16. http://www.dreamdoctors.org.il/en/Category/2/About_us
17. http://www.dreamdoctors.org.il/en/Pages/9/Research
18. http://www.dreamdoctors.org.il/en/Pages/17/Vision_and_Objectives
19. http://www.napkinrose.com/
20. http://www.ibtimes.com/miss-colorado-kelley-johnson-explains-why-she-chose-wear-nurse-uniform-miss-america-2103190
21. Dec 5-8, 2013 Gallup Poll
22. Mark Wilson. *Mark Wilson's Complete Course in Magic*. Running Press. Rev Ed (May 19, 2003). https://www.amazon.com/Mark-Wilsons-Complete-Course-Magic/dp/0762414553
23. Tokar, Scott and Harrison J Carroll. *Side-FX: Clinically*

Relevant Magic Effects and Tricks for the Health-Care Provider. Corporate-FX (2004). http://www.barnesandnoble.com/w/side-fx-scott-tokar/1006480431

24. Towsen, John H. *Clowns.* E P Dutton (Nov 1976). https://www.amazon.com/Clowns-John-H-Towsen/dp/0801539625

25. Simon, Eli. *The Art of Clowning.* Palgrave Macmillan (2009). https://www.amazon.com/Art-Clowning-Eli-Simon/dp/0230615236

26. Lecoq, Jacques, Jean-Gabriel Carasso, and Jean-Claude Lallias. Forward by Simon McBurney. *The Moving Body: Teaching Creative Theatre.* Routledge (Jan 2002). https://www.amazon.com/Moving-Body-Teaching-Creative-Theatre/dp/0878301410

27. Madson, Patricia Ryan. *Improv Wisdom: Don't Prepare, Just Show Up.* Bell Tower. 1st Ed (May 2005). https://www.amazon.com/dp/B003CIQ4XY/

28. Ocasio, Angel. *Clowning: Keep it Simple, Keep it Real.* http://www.ocomedy.com/a-clown-book

29. Dream, Caroline. *The Clown in You.* Alejandro Carlos Navarro Gonzalez. 1st Ed (June 2014). https://www.amazon.com/clown-you-Caroline-Dream/dp/8461696522